BLOOD
PRESSURE
DOWN

Also by Janet Bond Brill

Cholesterol Down
Prevent a Second Heart Attack

BLOOD PRESSURE DOWN

The 10-Step Plan to Lower Your Blood
Pressure in 4 Weeks—
Without Prescription Drugs

Janet Bond Brill, Ph.D., R.D., LDN

THREE RIVERS PRESS • NEW YORK

This book is not intended as a replacement for qualified, professional medical care. It is not intended to diagnose, prevent, treat, or cure any disease. Individuals with high blood pressure and/or those at risk for cardiovascular disease should first consult with their personal physician for medical clearance before making any of the dietary and lifestyle changes recommended in the Blood Pressure Down Plan. The Blood Pressure Down Plan should not be substituted for a physician-prescribed drug without the express permission of your personal physician. Blood pressure–lowering medications have been scientifically proven to lower the risk of death from cardiovascular disease and kidney disease whereas the Blood Pressure Down Plan has not yet been shown to prevent heart disease, heart attacks, stroke, or kidney disease. Several of the steps outlined may produce adverse reactions in some people and could potentially interact with over-the-counter and prescription medications. While every effort has been made to provide accurate and up-to-date information, this document cannot be guaranteed to be free of factual error. Consult your physician regarding applicability of any information provided in this book for your medical condition. The recipes are not intended for individuals prescribed special diets by their physician. Both the author and the publisher take no responsibility for any consequences that may arise from following the advice set forth within these pages.

Published in the United States by Three Rivers Press, an imprint of the Crown Publishing Group, a division of Random House, Inc., New York.

www.crownpublishing.com

Three Rivers Press and the Tugboat design are registered trademarks of Random House, Inc.

Library of Congress Cataloging-in-Publication Data
Brill, Janet Bond.
Blood pressure down : the 10-step plan to lower your blood pressure in 4 weeks—without prescription drugs / Janet Bond Brill, Ph.D., R.D., LDN.
Includes bibliographical references and index.
1. Hypertension—Alternative treatment.   2. Dietary supplements.
3. Physical fitness.   I. Title.
RC685.H8B75 2013
616.1'32—dc23   2012049634

ISBN 978-0-307-98635-1
eISBN 978-0-307-98636-8

Printed in the United States of America

Illustrations by Mia Alexandra Brill
Cover design by Deanna Destefano

10 9 8 7 6 5 4 3 2 1

First Edition

This book is dedicated to my brother, Zane Philip Bond,
who died of kidney disease and high blood pressure at the
young age of fifty-six. It is my hope that this book can potentially
prevent others from suffering his same fate.

To my dear mother, Dr. Alma Halbert Bond, this one's for you.

I also dedicate this book to my beloved husband, Sam,
who is always there for me in all ways that truly count.
Thank you and I love you.

And to my children, Rachel, Mia, and Jason, who are,
and always will be, my everything.

Contents

Foreword

Frequently called the "silent scourge," high blood pressure is as insidious as it is devastating. Almost invariably, it damages blood vessels silently—causing no pain, no discomfort, no symptoms—until disaster strikes in the form of a stroke, a weakened heart, a burst or dangerously dilated blood vessel, kidney failure, or a heart attack.

According to the most recent *Global Health Risks* report issued by the World Health Organization, high blood pressure is the leading global risk for mortality. Their research attributed to the condition a staggering annual death toll of 7.5 million, or more than one out of every eight of the world's deaths each year. In the United States, data from the National Health and Nutrition Examination Survey indicate that 67 million Americans—almost one-third of all U.S. adults—have high blood pressure, and of these, more than half have uncontrolled high blood pressure.

Fortunately, the battle against high blood pressure is not lost. I firmly believe you hold in your hands a critical component to winning your personal struggle with high blood pressure, as well as the greatest hope for defeating the epidemic we face as a society: *Blood Pressure Down*. Bringing her extensive experience as a dietitian, researcher, and author to bear on the prodigious problem of high blood pressure, Dr. Brill has created a scientifically rigorous, engaging, and practical guide to lowering your blood pressure through specific dietary, physical activity, and weight loss interventions. In doing so, she has distilled decades of research into an easy-to-read treatment program comprised of proven prescriptions for lifestyle changes that lower blood pressure. How effective are these measures? Consider that in one large, rigorously designed trial, over half of the people previously on a blood-pressure-lowering medication were able to stop taking their medication after weight loss and reduction of their salt intake—just two of the ten interventions detailed in this guide. Make no mistake: these changes work.

In a call to action, Centers for Disease Control and Prevention director Dr. Thomas Frieden charged the health care community to make high blood pressure "a priority for every doctor's visit." In the same vein, I urge you to prioritize the daily choices you make about your diet and physical activity in order to improve your blood pressure and overall health. I urge you to read this book and to heed Dr. Brill's evidence-based recommendations.

—EMIL M. deGOMA, M.D.
Medical Director, Preventive Cardiovascular Program
Division of Cardiovascular Medicine
University of Pennsylvania

Acknowledgments

Writing a book is always a collaborative process. I am thrilled to give credit where credit is due and to have this opportunity to thank the many people who helped make *Blood Pressure Down* a reality.

First, I would like to thank my longtime literary agent, Faith Hamlin, for giving me that little extra push to get this idea into words and a concrete proposal. I also owe a debt of gratitude to my cousin, Zachary Dreier, who inspired me to write on this topic. Thank you to my fantastic editor at Three Rivers Press, Anna Thompson. I was fortunate enough to work with Anna on my second book, *Prevent a Second Heart Attack*, so naturally I was delighted that Anna was assigned as my editor for *Blood Pressure Down*. Anna is such a pleasure to work with. She is truly a dream editor whose professional expertise effortlessly shaped and polished the manuscript. This book simply would not have been possible without her professional guidance.

I am indebted to my dietitian colleague, Maggie Green, who helped formulate and test the myriad recipes. Creating delicious recipes without sodium is truly an artistic endeavor. I would also like to extend my gratitude to another dietitian colleague, Caitlin Riley. Caitlin provided factual nutrition data and menu creation, thereby giving me the freedom to focus more on writing and research rather than on calculations.

I am honored to thank the highly esteemed Emil M. deGoma, M.D., assistant professor of medicine at the Hospital of the University of Pennsylvania and medical director of the Preventive Cardiovascular Program of the Division of Cardiovascular Medicine at the Perelman Center for Advanced Medicine in Philadelphia, for his significant contribution to this book. As I am not a medical expert, I am deeply grateful to Dr. deGoma for agreeing to read and comment on the medical aspects of the initial manuscript as well as writing such a wonderfully informative foreword to this book.

To my "other" parents, Edna and Harry Brill—kind and generous in-laws—thank you for raising (and giving me) your incredibly supportive and simply amazing son! Finally, I would like to thank our dear friends for their encouragement and support. To Ellen and Arthur Fein, Brian and Lynn Berkowitz, Dr. Bob Bergen (thanks for the medical information on the human eye!) and Cheryl Bergen, Abbe and Marc Sloven, and wonderful new friends, Ramzi Haddad and Dr. Anita Shrivastava—I love you all.

Introduction

Chances are you're reading this book because you or someone you love has high blood pressure. I too have been affected personally by this insidious disease. My grandmother died of a stroke when I was just six months old. My brother died prematurely, at age fifty-six, from kidney failure due to complications of high blood pressure. Cardiovascular disease runs in my family; my father had his first heart attack at forty-five and died several years later from a second heart attack. He too had high blood pressure.

It is my grandmother's, brother's, and father's untimely deaths from this insidious disease that have inspired me to write with great passion about cardiovascular disease (CVD) prevention through simple lifestyle changes. CVD is far and away our nation's leading cause of death, and high blood pressure is the main contributing factor for its development. Heart attacks disable or kill men in their forties and fifties, during their most productive years. And while women take a decade to catch up to men, heart attacks and stroke are the leading causes of death for them too. *High blood pressure contributes to more deaths in men and women than any other preventable factor.*[1] But the good news is, it can easily be controlled. I hope that this book will help others suffering from high blood pressure to avoid the fate of my grandmother, father, and brother.

If you already have high blood pressure and your doctor has

prescribed medication, be sure to take it as directed. But it's important to know that there are also ways to lower your blood pressure naturally. As a health professional specializing in using a natural lifestyle approach (diet and exercise, also called *lifestyle therapy*) to treat and prevent cardiovascular disease, I have found that many of my patients are averse to taking prescription medications to control their blood pressure. Most are fully aware of the danger of high blood pressure. But perhaps they have had intolerable side effects, or they hate the idea of taking a drug every day for the rest of their lives.

My message in this book is that high blood pressure is the most preventable cause of premature morbidity and mortality in the United States and the world, and that lifestyle therapy is the cornerstone of treatment for this disease. Unfortunately, many people are confused by the myriad recommendations, some have difficulty following tasteless low-sodium diets, and others are overwhelmed by the plethora of complicated self-help plans that crowd the bookstore shelves. Time and again, my patients ask me for a simple, doable lifestyle plan that will get their blood pressure down, quickly and safely. This book is just that. It is a book about taking charge of your blood pressure. Follow the simple steps set forth in these pages and you will surely transform your life, your health, and your future.

Why focus on lifestyle therapy when effective prescription drugs are available? You should know that all health professionals are advised by the medical community to actively promote lifestyle strategies *first and foremost* as the basis for controlling blood pressure and preventing CVD. A drug alone is simply not enough. If all health care providers promoted healthy living as the foundation for treatment, we would have a cost-effective and practical means of helping to solve our country's blood pressure epidemic and improve health and longevity. Sad to say, though, few doctors have the time or expertise to teach their patients the modest lifestyle changes that would help them.

The lifestyle strategies outlined in the Blood Pressure Down program, alone or in concert with prescription medications, have the potential to lower blood pressure, enhance the effectiveness of blood pressure medications, and promote health in your arteries. What are the side effects of the Blood Pressure Down plan? Weight loss, more energy, and a happier and healthier cardiovascular system . . . not too bad a payoff for taking charge of your lifestyle!

The U.S. government agrees. Lifestyle therapy to reduce blood pressure is recommended in *The Seventh Report of the Joint National Committee on Prevention, Detection, Evaluation, and Treatment of High Blood Pressure* (or JNC 7) as the first line of therapy for the prevention of high blood pressure, and in combination with medication for the optimal management of diagnosed high blood pressure and its health consequences.

There are indeed powerful drugs available that can quickly and effectively lower your blood pressure. This method of treatment is great for doctors (write a prescription, get patient results fast) and for drug companies (huge sales). Drugs save millions of lives in the United States today, and many have excellent safety records. But half of all blood pressure drug prescriptions are left unfilled. Why? For some patients, the medications are prohibitively expensive. Others fear the notorious list of potential side effects.

Perhaps you are not ready to hop on the prescription bandwagon just yet. Or maybe you are willing to try a lifestyle plan alongside your prescribed medication; once you're successful, your doctor may cut your dosage or even allow you to move to a lifestyle-only long-term plan. I encourage you to try this inexpensive, safe, and scientifically sound natural approach that takes advantage of artery-friendly minerals such as potassium and calcium, cuts down on artery-damaging sodium, and adds in exercise such as brisk walking, which has been proven to produce impressive blood pressure reductions. Yes, there is a better way—a healthier, drug-free plan for lowering blood pressure without any side effects.

BLOOD PRESSURE DRUGS: WHAT ARE THE SIDE EFFECTS?

It is estimated that patients typically take only 50–70 percent of the medication prescribed for them. This high noncompliance rate is often attributed to the fact that some individuals experience intolerable side effects from taking blood-pressure-lowering drugs. Here is a list of the most commonly reported undesirable side effects:

- Fatigue, drowsiness, sedation, lethargy
- Sexual dysfunction
- Cough
- Depression
- Dry mouth
- Weakness
- Headache, dizziness
- Insomnia
- Gout
- Heart and/or kidney dysfunction

Sources: Alhalaiqa F, et al. Adherence therapy for medication non-compliant patients with hypertension: a randomized controlled trial. *J Hum Hypertens* 2012;26:117–126; Moser M. Antihypertensive medications: relative effectiveness and adverse reactions. *J Hypertens* 2011;8(Suppl 2):S9–S16; Rosenfeldt FL, Haas SJ, Krum H, et al. Coenzyme Q10 in the treatment of hypertension: a meta-analysis of the clinical trials. *J Hum Hypertens* 2007;21(4):297–306.

In response to my patients' requests for blood-pressure-lowering techniques that didn't involve drugs, I began doing extensive research and decided to develop a diet and exercise prescription for reducing blood pressure, based on sound science. The result is a mixture of foods and exercise scientifically proven to effectively lower blood pressure. I was amazed to discover that several of these lifestyle modifications could reduce blood pressure as much as a starting dose of a blood pressure drug.

This safe and easy-to-follow plan is built on the concept of combining numerous lifestyle approaches to achieve an additive effect. Individually, each step has been scientifically proven to lower blood pressure a few millimeters. By itself, that may seem tiny—but when several steps are taken together, the results are nothing short of miraculous.

WHO SHOULD GO ON THIS PLAN

I designed this plan for healthy adults who either are interested in preventing the onset of high blood pressure or have diagnosed high blood pressure and want to lower it using a safe and effective drug-free approach. The Blood Pressure Down plan is also ideal for people who are already taking prescription blood pressure drugs. By using my plan to supplement their blood pressure medication, they can keep their dosages low enough to reduce the risk of side effects. As an adjunct to medication, the Blood Pressure Down plan can be very effective for those with stubbornly high blood pressure who are having difficulty attaining their blood pressure goal.

HOW TO USE THIS BOOK

There are two main parts to this book. Part I (Chapters One through Three) provides the scientific background for the Blood Pressure Down plan. You'll learn everything you need to know about high blood pressure, how you got it, and what can happen if you don't control it. I have included many scientific references for those especially interested in the latest research findings. If science is not your cup of tea, simply skip to Part II, the plan itself, to start bringing your blood pressure down now.

Part II (Chapters Four through Thirteen) lays out the ten steps of the Blood Pressure Down plan. Before you begin, I suggest you read all the steps, and pay particular attention to the caveats at the end of certain chapters. After getting the go-ahead from your physician, begin by assessing your starting point: take your pressure by following the instructions in Chapter One. You can purchase a highly affordable home blood pressure monitoring machine at your local pharmacy; just make sure it is accurate by comparing it to readings at your doctor's office. You will need to test your blood pressure every day, twice a day (same time and place), for at least four weeks to track your progress.

Make several photocopies of the Ten-Step Daily Checklist (see Appendix 2), purchase all the components (the blood pressure monitor, the food, the supplements, a scale, and a pair of sneakers if need be), and you're ready to begin. Checking off your daily steps will help you get in all ten every day. The appendixes provide tools for helping you stick to the Blood Pressure Down plan. In addition

---

BENEFITS OF LOWERING BLOOD PRESSURE: WHAT'S IN IT FOR YOU?

There is an enormous, ever-growing body of scientific research supporting the health benefits of lowering elevated blood pressure. One thing is certain: high blood pressure, if left uncontrolled, has severe health consequences down the road, including stroke, heart attack, and heart failure. Getting your blood pressure down dramatically reduces your risk of these diseases. According to the JNC 7, lowering your blood pressure will:

- Reduce your odds of having a stroke by 35–40 percent
- Reduce your odds of having a heart attack by 20–25 percent
- Reduce your odds of heart failure by 50 percent

The steps in the Blood Pressure Down plan will help lower your blood pressure for maximum disease protection.

Source: National High Blood Pressure Education Program. *The Seventh Report of the Joint National Committee on Prevention, Detection, Evaluation, and Treatment of High Blood Pressure.* Bethesda, MD: National Heart, Lung, and Blood Institute; 2004.

to the Ten-Step Daily Checklist, there are Blood Pressure and Body Weight Progress Charts (Appendixes 2 and 4), two weeks of sample menus (Appendix 7), and more than fifty heart-healthy recipes incorporating the required foods in the plan (Appendix 8). Make four photocopies of your weekly blood pressure progress chart and you will be ready to get your blood pressure down!

Know Your Numbers and Count Your Way to Better Health

It's a numbers game! Ultimately, your key statistics are a reflection of your health. Make an appointment with your primary care physician and have him or her help you fill in the numbers. Here are the six vital numbers you need to know:

1. Blood pressure (millimeters of mercury, or mm HG): aim for under 120/80
2. Body weight: aim for a body mass index (BMI) of 25 or less
3. Bad cholesterol (LDL) (milligrams per deciliter, or mg/dL): aim for under 100
4. Good cholesterol (HDL) (mg/dL): aim for over 40 (over 60 is even better)
5. Triglyceride (mg/dL): aim for under 150
6. Fasting blood sugar (mg/dL): aim for under 100

You have the power to manipulate these six numbers and ultimately control your health. In this book, we will tackle your blood pressure and your body weight. To change these numbers, you will need to utilize some basic arithmetic and keep track of six more numbers. So get out those calculators! We will be accounting daily for these numbers:

1. Body weight (recorded weekly) and calorie intake (recorded daily)

2. Salt (sodium) intake: less than 1,500 mg daily
3. Potassium intake: at least 4,700 mg daily
4. Magnesium intake: at least 500 mg daily
5. Calcium intake: at least 1,200 mg daily
6. Soy protein: at least 25 g daily

If counting is simply not for you, then just stick to the daily checklist, eat and exercise as prescribed, and watch those portion sizes. You will be taking a giant leap toward getting your blood pressure down.

HOW THIS BOOK DIFFERS FROM OTHER BLOOD PRESSURE BOOKS

Every good lifestyle program for lowering blood pressure should incorporate a DASH-type diet—the only diet scientifically proven to lower blood pressure. (DASH stands for Dietary Approaches to Stop Hypertension.) There are plenty of books on the market that outline how to follow the DASH diet. What these books *don't* give you are the numerous additional steps that have also been scientifically shown to reduce blood pressure. *Blood Pressure Down* is unique in that it incorporates *all* of the lifestyle factors proven to lower blood pressure, combined into one simple yet highly potent program. I'll give you a clear, step-by-step plan outlining exactly what foods to eat and in what amounts, and how to exercise and how much. I also explain the scientific basis behind each step so that you understand why the plan works and how each step lowers blood pressure in a different way for the maximum cumulative effect. I ask you to devote just four weeks of your life to this plan, to develop new habits and track your dropping pressure. It is my hope that when you see the results after four weeks—lower blood pressure, a lower body weight, and a new sense of vitality—you will embrace these new habits for the rest of your life. In doing so, you may even save your life.

Blood Pressure Down is the culmination of my experience as a registered and licensed dietitian, exercise physiologist, and certified wellness coach. The plan is user-friendly and designed to make it easy for you to stay on track. I hope that this book will be a powerful, potentially lifesaving tool for you and the millions of Americans who want a safer, natural alternative or supplement to blood pressure drugs for getting your blood pressure down.

Part I

Everything You Need to Know About High Blood Pressure and Your Health

Understanding the Problem

The doctor of the future will give no medicine, but will interest his patients in the care of the human body, in diet, and in the cause and prevention of disease.

—Thomas Alva Edison

LOOSENING THE GRIP OF HIGH BLOOD PRESSURE

Why do so many people in this country have high blood pressure? What triggers the squeeze on the arteries that puts you at grave risk for heart disease and stroke, the first- and third-leading causes of death in the United States?

We used to think that high blood pressure was an inevitable consequence of aging. But in recent decades, research has revealed a surprising truth: high blood pressure doesn't have to be a by-product of getting older. It is a lifestyle-borne illness that is more related to our daily habits than to our biological clock. A toxic mix of calorie overload—especially from processed foods high in salt, sugars, and damaging fats—inactivity, and middle-aged spread instigates the rising squeeze on the arteries, a relentless pressure cooker that eventually injures the fragile cells that line our inner arterial walls, causing irreparable and life-threatening damage. The good news? All this means that high blood pressure can be prevented and treated.

In the chapters that follow, you will discover how, when, and why your blood pressure began to rise. You will then learn about the exciting world of nonmedicinal approaches to lowering blood pressure and how you can take control of your blood pressure the Blood Pressure Down way. These tools will allow you to conquer high blood pressure, reverse the course of your disease, and ultimately protect yourself against heart attacks and stroke—the most likely end product of years of uncontrolled high blood pressure—for many decades to come.

America's Blood Pressure Burden

If you have been diagnosed with high blood pressure, you are certainly not alone. The number of Americans who have high blood pressure has risen sharply in the past few decades. According to the most recent Centers for Disease Control and Prevention estimate, more than 76 million adult Americans—about one-third of the population—suffer from this life-threatening condition. Early high blood pressure, which is also known as prehypertension and describes a blood pressure measurement that is higher than normal but not yet in the high blood pressure range, afflicts an additional one-third of adult Americans. In fact, new survey data show that approximately 70 percent of adult Americans have an unhealthy blood pressure level (34 percent have full-blown hypertension and 36 percent have prehypertension).[1] The incidence of high blood pressure rises with age, such that more than half of all Americans sixty-five and older have the condition. This disease damages not only our nation's health but also our wallets: high blood pressure is estimated to cost the United States approximately $74 billion in health care services, medications, and missed days of work annually. Of all the cardiovascular diseases (high blood pressure, heart disease, heart failure, and stroke), hypertension is the most expensive, with annual costs projected to increase to $200 billion by the year 2030.[2]

HIGH BLOOD PRESSURE BY THE NUMBERS

- One in three adults (more than 76 million Americans) has high blood pressure (and this number is likely even higher, as high blood pressure is asymptomatic).
- One in three adults with high blood pressure (approximately 23 million Americans) is not even aware he or she has the disease.
- One in two adults with high blood pressure is not being treated effectively, hence does not have his or her high blood pressure under control.
- An additional 30 percent of the adult population in the United States has an early form of the disease known as prehypertension.
- High blood pressure prevalence is nearly equal between men and women until the older age groups (over age fifty-five), where women have a higher prevalence.
- Approximately 60 percent of white women over age forty-five have high blood pressure. For African American women, the number is even higher—79 percent.
- At 44 percent, African American adults have one of the highest rates of high blood pressure in the world.

The takeaway message? There are millions of Americans walking around with uncontrolled disease that puts them at great risk for dire health consequences and premature death.

Sources: American Heart Association. Heart disease and stroke statistics—2012 update. *Circulation* 2012;125:e2–e220; Danaei G, Ding EL, Mozaffarian D, et al. The preventable causes of death in the United States: comparative risk assessment of dietary, lifestyle, and metabolic risk factors. *PLoS Med* 2009;6(4):e1000058. DOI:10.1371/journal .pmed.1000058.

What Is Hypertension?

Hypertension is the medical term for high blood pressure. It is an extraordinarily common cardiovascular disease (CVD) in the United States. In fact, it is the most widespread chronic disease in Western society. Despite major medical advances in the understanding and treatment of high blood pressure over the past several decades, the disease remains the most common medical diagnosis in the United States and the condition that doctors write the most prescriptions for. It is also the number one cause of stroke and kidney disease and a principal cause of heart disease and blindness. High blood pressure ranks among the most powerful risk factors for developing CVD and accounts for about 30 percent of all cardiovascular events (primarily heart attacks or stroke). No wonder your doctor is so concerned! Blood pressure is the vital sign that doctors monitor most often and treat most aggressively. And rightly so—in simple terms, walking around with untreated high blood pressure makes you a ticking time bomb, liable to suffer a heart attack or stroke.

You should also know that the odds are very good that you will die from some form of CVD—our nation's deadliest epidemic. In the United States, one person dies from CVD approximately every thirty-nine seconds.[3] Combine that overwhelming death toll with the staggering direct cost to the global health care system of more than $500 billion annually and you will begin to grasp the magnitude of this huge public health concern.[4]

High blood pressure is also known as the "silent killer" because it is a largely symptomless disease. This is what makes high blood pressure so insidious: you can't see or feel it, yet if it is left untreated, it will kill you. It is no wonder that 8 percent of the adult U.S. population has undiagnosed high blood pressure—they can't feel that anything is wrong. Perhaps this is one reason that, of the over 76 million adult Americans already diagnosed with high blood pressure, a whopping 56 percent do not have it under control. If you are one of the people who believes that if there was really a problem you would feel it, think again. You are taking a chance with your life. The fact is, the higher your numbers and the longer you have uncontrolled high blood pressure, the greater your risk of developing the devastating health consequences that often accompany high blood pressure—all the more reason for you to find out your numbers and start today to get your blood pressure down.

A NATION UNDER PRESSURE: THE DIRE CONSEQUENCES

According to the most recent research estimates:

- High blood pressure was directly responsible for one in six deaths in 2005.
- High blood pressure is the single largest risk factor for death from heart attack or stroke—responsible for almost half of all cardiovascular deaths.
- From 1995 to 2005, the death rate from high blood pressure rose by 25 percent.
- In 2009, high blood pressure cost our nation approximately $73 billion (direct and indirect costs).
- Nearly 400,000 deaths occur each year directly attributed to high blood pressure.
- Every thirty-nine seconds an American dies from a heart attack or stroke.
- Seventy-seven percent of first-time stroke victims have high blood pressure.
- Sixty-nine percent of first-time heart attack victims have high blood pressure.
- Seventy-four percent of first-time heart failure victims have high blood pressure.

Sources: Institute of Medicine. *Strategies to Reduce Sodium Intake in the United States.* Washington, DC: National Academies Press; 2010; American Heart Association. Heart disease and stroke statistics—2012 update. *Circulation* 2012;125:e2–e220.

Prolong Your Life, Preserve Your Health

The good news is that high blood pressure is one of the few risk factors for cardiovascular disease that is recognized as reversible.

Scientific studies have proven that getting your blood pressure under control will preserve your health.[5] High blood pressure is a lifestyle disease. So modifying your lifestyle is your most powerful protection against diseases of the heart and blood vessels. Healthy lifestyle modifications (exercise, consuming certain foods, and reducing intake of other foods) have proven to be the most effective medicine both for preventing new-onset high blood pressure and for reducing diagnosed high blood pressure quickly and safely.

A GLOBAL HEALTH CRISIS

Worldwide, high blood pressure strikes hard. It has been estimated that more than a billion people have high blood pressure, making high blood pressure responsible for the greatest number of preventable deaths on this earth. According to the International Society of Hypertension, elevated blood pressure is responsible for 7.6 million premature deaths each year. Of all the heart attacks and strokes around the globe, most are attributed to high blood pressure—with half of those surfacing in people with prehypertension (early high blood pressure). According to the World Health Organization, high blood pressure is the most prevalent risk factor for heart attacks and stroke, with high blood pressure affecting about 20 percent of the entire global adult population. (It is projected that by the year 2025, this number will rise to 29 percent, or over 1.5 billion adults.)

Sources: Lawes CMM, Vander Hoorn SV, Rodgers A, for the International Society of Hypertension. Global burden of blood-pressure-related disease, 2001. *Lancet* 2008;371:1513–1518; World Health Organization. Cardiovascular diseases. www.who .int/topics/cardiovascular_diseases/en; Kearney PM, et al. Global burden of hypertension: analysis of worldwide data. *Lancet* 2005;365:217–223; World Health Organization. Global health risks: mortality and burden of disease attributable to selected major risks. www.who.int/healthinfo/global_burden_disease/GlobalHealthRisks_report_full.pdf

---

What Do the Blood Pressure Numbers Mean?

Your blood pressure is one of the main vital signs, or measures of your physiology, that give your health care provider a picture of your general state of health. (Other vital signs typically include your heart rate, body temperature, and respiratory rate.) But what do the numbers mean? The heart is a muscle with the primary function of pumping blood. When the heart beats, it pumps blood around the large network of blood vessels in your body, and it must create pressure to propel the blood. The term *blood pressure* (also known as *systemic blood pressure*) typically refers to the pressure in the arteries, excluding those between the heart and lungs. (This is different from *pulmonary blood pressure*, which refers to the pressure in the specific arteries circulating blood between the heart and the lungs.) Your blood pressure normally rises when the heart beats—when blood is being propelled out from the heart into the aorta or main artery—and falls when the heart relaxes.

More specifically, the systemic pressure is actually the result of two forces. The first, the systolic pressure, is the force of the blood on the artery walls as it is ejected out of the heart. The second is the diastolic pressure, the pressure in your arteries when the heart rests between beats and is refilling with blood. Blood pressure is therefore written as two numbers. The top number is the systolic pressure—the peak pressure in the arteries. The bottom number is the diastolic pressure—the lowest pressure in the arteries, which occurs near the beginning of the cardiac cycle. Your blood pressure reading is expressed as a ratio of these two numbers, and is always written as systolic (top number) over diastolic (bottom number). A reading of 140/90 mm Hg, for example, means your systolic blood pressure is 140 mm Hg (the peak pressure in your arteries) and your diastolic pressure is 90 mm Hg (the pressure in your arteries when your heart is at rest, between beats).

How Low Can You Go?

Your blood pressure changes throughout the day depending on many factors, including activity level, stress, sleep, and exercise. If you have a low blood pressure reading (defined as a reading less than

90 systolic or less than 60 diastolic), great. There is no day-to-day pressure that is considered too low unless there are noticeable symptoms such as dizziness, fainting, or excessive fatigue. This would alert your physician to a potential problem that needs to be remedied, often by lowering the dosage of certain medications. In rare instances, unusually low pressure could also be a sign of a serious illness, so be sure to check with your doctor.

WHAT IS NORMAL AND SAFE?

According to the American Heart Association, healthy adults should have a blood pressure reading of less than 120 mm Hg systolic *and* less than 80 mm Hg diastolic. It is estimated that one in three American adults has an unhealthy blood pressure level.

Blood pressure is measured in millimeters of mercury (mm Hg). Why mercury? The gold standard of blood pressure measurement devices has always been the sphygmomanometer (pronounced "sfig-moh-muh-nom-i-ter"). This device has been around for decades and historically used the height of a column of mercury to assess the two blood pressure values. Newer blood pressure measurement devices such as aneroid and electronic gauges do not use mercury, but we still use the millimeters of mercury measurement.

What Defines High Blood Pressure?

Your doctor's "bible" of blood pressure diagnoses and treatment guidelines is *The Seventh Report of the Joint National Committee on Prevention, Detection, Evaluation, and Treatment of High Blood Pressure.*[6] Written by a prestigious group of doctors and scientists from a variety of professional, public, and voluntary organizations and federal agencies, the JNC 7 is the definitive, most up-to-date set of guidelines for the diagnosis and treatment of high blood pressure. The JNC 7 defines normal blood pressure as a top number (systolic) of less than 120 mm Hg and a bottom number (diastolic) of less than 80 mm Hg.

The Two Highs of High Blood Pressure

High blood pressure occurs in two forms, primary and secondary. *Primary* (also called *essential*) is the most common—from 90 percent to 95 percent of all the people diagnosed with high blood pressure fall under this classification. Primary high blood pressure means that the direct cause for the condition is unknown. It could be due to any number of factors, such as sedentary lifestyle, obesity, high salt intake, or aging. Other risk factors for essential high blood pressure are an overactive nervous system and too much renin, a hormone secreted by the kidney that constricts blood vessel diameter.

Secondary high blood pressure directly results from an identifiable cause—another disease or disorder such as sleep apnea, hyperaldosteronism, kidney disease, Cushing's syndrome, hyperthyroidism, or high-dose estrogen therapy. Secondary high blood pressure is often suspected in younger individuals hospitalized for high blood pressure, in highly resistant hypertension, or in people who have had a sudden rise in blood pressure that has been previously controlled. Fewer than 5 percent of diagnosed cases of high blood pressure fall under this classification. The treatment for secondary high blood pressure varies, as the physician must treat the underlying condition.

The Blood Pressure Down plan is designed to treat both classes of high blood pressure, keeping in mind that the second type requires additional medical intervention to address the causative problem. In many cases, if the triggering medical issue is fixed, so is the high blood pressure.

Regardless of which form of high blood pressure you have, the dangers are the same. High blood pressure increases your risk of blood vessel and organ damage, which, if left untreated, leads to complications down the road such as kidney failure, stroke, and heart attack. The longer you wait and the higher your numbers, the higher your risks.

The Latest Government Blood Pressure Guidelines: What You Need to Know

The latest version of the JNC 7 was published in 2003 (albeit at the time of this writing, the release of the newest version, JNC 8, was imminent) and contained some key updates that you should know about:

- The prehypertension (early high blood pressure) category was introduced. As noted previously, people with blood pressure at the high end of what was once a normal reading fall into this class. Starting at 115/75 mm Hg, risk for cardiovascular disease doubles with each increment of 20/10 mm Hg, which is why a classification of prehypertension is cause for concern.
- When people develop high blood pressure at a relatively young age (under fifty), it's typically the bottom number that is too high. For people over fifty, however, it's the top number, or systolic blood pressure, that can really climb. This is much more worrisome than an elevated bottom number. Why? Because as we age, the arteries close to the heart begin to stiffen, increasing the workload of the heart as it pushes blood through. This scenario strains the heart muscle and increases risk of plaque buildup in the coronary arteries (a precursor to a heart attack). So in older people, the top number—which tells us how hard the heart has to work—reflects the risk of CVD more accurately than the bottom number. Medically, this phenomenon of high systolic pressure with a normal diastolic pressure is termed *isolated systolic hypertension*.

- People who have normal blood pressure at age fifty-five are not out of the woods yet—they still have a 90 percent lifetime risk for developing high blood pressure.

NUMBERS YOUR DOCTOR WILL BE CONCERNED ABOUT

- **Prehypertension.** The following numbers categorize you as having prehypertension: systolic blood pressure (top number) of 120 to 139 mm Hg or diastolic blood pressure (bottom number) of 80 to 89 mm Hg. It is estimated that 15 percent of deaths from heart attacks occur in people with blood pressure in the prehypertension range. *Individuals with prehypertension face twice the risk of developing full-blown hypertension compared to those whose blood pressure is normal.*
- **Stage 1 hypertension.** Systolic blood pressure (top number) of 140 to 159 mm Hg or diastolic blood pressure (bottom number) of 90 to 99 mm Hg. *Individuals with stage 1 hypertension are advised by the JNC 7 to take a prescription medication (typically a thiazide diuretic)—in addition to lifestyle therapy—to treat their hypertension.*
- **Stage 2 hypertension.** Systolic blood pressure (top number) of 160 mm Hg or more or diastolic blood pressure (bottom number) of 100 mm Hg or more. *Individuals with stage 2 hypertension are advised by the JNC 7 to take at least a two-drug prescription medication combination—in addition to lifestyle therapy—to treat their high blood pressure. Side effects pose significant problems for these people, associated with increasing doses and increasing numbers of medications. Medication cost can also be a problem.*

Sources: National High Blood Pressure Education Program. The seventh report of the Joint National Committee on Prevention, Detection, Evaluation, and Treatment of High Blood Pressure. *Hypertens* 2003;42:1206–1252; Jones DW, et al. The effect of weight loss intervention on antihypertensive medication requirements in the Hypertension Optimal Treatment (HOT) study. *Am J Hypertens* 1999;12:1175–1180.

Fortunately, there are a number of simple lifestyle changes that can loosen the grip of all forms of high blood pressure and protect your arteries. In future chapters, you will use the Blood Pressure Down plan to dramatically lower your blood pressure numbers and reduce your chances of developing cardiovascular disease, including atherosclerosis—the clogging of the arteries with plaque—which is the cause of most heart attacks and strokes.

DO YOU REALLY HAVE HIGH BLOOD PRESSURE?

One elevated blood pressure reading, even by a trained physician, is not enough to diagnose high blood pressure. Although blood pressure measurements are probably the most important clinical assessment in all of medicine, they are notoriously inaccurate. There are many reasons for this: some measurement devices or techniques are simply not precise enough; blood pressure varies throughout the day—for example, it goes up with stress or after a meal; and some people's pressure shoots up in the presence of a health care worker.[7]

To ensure an accurate reading, the measurement should always be taken after you have been sitting calmly for five minutes. Have the physician take multiple readings. In fact, new research suggests that it is best to have your health care provider take measurements in both arms. If there is a consistent difference of at least 20 mm Hg systolic (top number) or 10 mm Hg diastolic (bottom number), then use the arm with the higher pressure for decision making. You need to measure both arms to diagnose and treat hypertension accurately—a consistent blood pressure difference of more than 20/10 mm Hg may indicate a greater cardiovascular risk and the need for more aggressive treatment.[8] If your numbers are high in the doctor's office, measure your pressure yourself in a calm environment using the home monitor discussed later in this chapter.

MEASURING BLOOD PRESSURE

Your blood pressure can be measured in three locations: the arm, the wrist, and the finger. You have probably had it taken in the upper arm, which is the most common site. (Note that finger monitors are inaccurate and not recommended.) Currently, there are three main techniques used to measure your blood pressure: the sphygmomanometer, the ambulatory monitor, and the home monitor.

Measurement Technique Number One:
The Sphygmomanometer

The first method takes place in your doctor's office and often involves the use of a mercury blood pressure gauge called a *sphygmomanometer*. The mercury sphygmomanometer consists of the cuff that encircles your arm, a tube that attaches to the cuff, and the thermometer-like column of mercury—the blood pressure gauge (Figure 1.1). When the cuff is inflated with air (by squeezing the rubber ball attached to it), it cuts off blood flow in the artery. A trained technician then listens with a stethoscope to five different

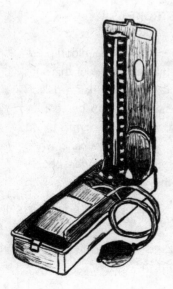

Figure 1.1 The sphygmomanometer, used by a trained health professional in a doctor's office, has always been regarded as the gold standard of blood pressure measurement techniques. The mercury within the gauge reflects the amount of pressure, with the numbers along the column of mercury indicating the reading.

types of sound coming from the artery, recording the mercury readings at each sound. For this reason, the sphygmomanometer is also called an *auscultation* (listening) technique.

Chances are you've had this done at the doctor's office, but you may not have understood what was going on. The technician inflates the cuff to a pressure that exceeds your systolic blood pressure; at this point, blood flow is totally occluded and there is no audible sound. (Think of a garden hose with water in it that is being clamped shut.) The technician then slowly releases pressure on the cuff until a tapping noise is heard. This is called the *first Korotkoff sound* and is the sound of the blood starting to rush back into and through the slightly opened artery. The number on the mercury column at that moment is your systolic blood pressure. As the pressure in the cuff falls further, additional sounds are heard. Eventually the cuff no longer restricts blood flow at all—the blood can flow smoothly through the artery—and so the sounds disappear altogether. This silence is known as the *fifth Korotkoff sound*, and

---

EVEN SLIGHTLY HIGH BLOOD PRESSURE
UPS YOUR ODDS OF STROKE

Not too concerned about your slightly higher than normal blood pressure readings? Findings from a new study may change your thinking. A recent review of twelve studies including more than half a million people found that those with prehypertension had a 55 percent increased risk of having a stroke compared to adults with normal blood pressure. And youth does not protect you. Even more dramatic, when researchers isolated data from middle-aged and younger people (under age sixty-five), it was found that the younger subjects with prehypertension had a 68 percent increased risk of stroke compared with those of the same age group with normal readings.

Source: Lee M, Saver JL, Chang B, et al. Presence of baseline prehypertension and risk of incident stroke: a meta-analysis. *Neurology* 2011. Sept 28.

the number on the mercury column at this point is your diastolic blood pressure.

The use of mercury devices is declining due to health and environmental concerns. Because mercury is highly toxic for humans, animals, and the ecosystem, some doctors use mercury-free electronic devices such as the aneroid sphygmomanometer, which uses air pressure to move a needle on a circular scale and does not require listening to the sounds coming from the artery. Aneroid blood pressure gauges are increasing in popularity, but they require frequent calibration and have been shown to be less accurate than mercury sphygmomanometers.

Measurement Technique Number Two: The Ambulatory Monitor

The second technique that your doctor may suggest involves a portable electronic device called an *ambulatory blood pressure monitor*, which consists of a cuff that attaches to the arm and then to a machine. You may have encountered one of these if you've ever been hospitalized. The cuff automatically inflates and takes a reading approximately every half hour during the day, and every hour or so during the night. The data are then stored in a computer, which allows your doctor to assess your typical blood pressure pattern over an entire day.

This technique is valuable because it helps detect "nondippers"— people whose pressure remains elevated at night (most people's blood pressure drops while they sleep). Nondippers are at greater risk of death from heart attacks or stroke than "dippers." Ambulatory blood pressure monitors can also determine if you have what is called *white coat syndrome*, where blood pressure surges at the doctor's office in response to anxiety but is lower at home.[9]

Measurement Technique Number Three: The Do-It-Yourself Home Monitor

The last technique involves purchasing your own electronic blood pressure machine and taking measurements yourself. These devices are safe, affordable, and widely available. The electronic machines measure your blood pressure at the upper arm or wrist; all you need to do is put the cuff on and press a button to inflate it. The machine then measures the pressure and uses an algorithm to estimate your numbers, and the screen provides you with a reading. While these machines are quite effective, you must ensure that yours is giving you an accurate reading before you begin using it. Take your machine in to your doctor and compare readings with his or her sphygmomanometer (and do this every six months).

Measuring your own blood pressure in a quiet and comfortable home setting can empower you to get your blood pressure under control. It provides you with a mirror, reflecting in measurable numbers how your new healthy lifestyle is affecting your body. If a single blood pressure reading is a movie still, multiple readings, tracked and recorded regularly, constitute a full-length feature film

WHEN TO CALL 911

If your blood pressure is severely elevated—over 180 systolic (top number) or over 110 diastolic (bottom number)—call 911 immediately. A high blood pressure crisis reflects either a hypertensive urgency situation, without associated organ damage, or a hypertensive emergency, which means organ damage is occurring. *A hypertensive emergency requires immediate emergency medical assistance.*

Stroke, a much feared complication of high blood pressure, also requires immediate medical attention. An acronym that will help you to remember what the common symptoms of a stroke are is **FAST:**

> **F**acial droop
> **A**rm weakness
> **S**lurred speech
> **T**ime—get to the hospital quickly!

HOME BLOOD PRESSURE MEASUREMENT INSTRUCTIONS

Take control of your health and learn how to obtain an accurate blood pressure reading at home so that you can monitor your progress over the next four weeks. Record the readings on the Blood Pressure Progress Chart in Appendix 4.

INSTRUCTIONS
- Make sure the blood pressure monitor has the correct size cuff before you buy it.
- Ensure your home blood pressure monitor is accurate by taking it into your doctor's office every six months and comparing the results with a mercury blood pressure gauge.
- Take your blood pressure twice a day, at the same times each day, morning and evening.
- Don't smoke, drink caffeine or alcohol, or perform any exercise within fifteen minutes of measuring your blood pressure.
- Rest five minutes before taking your blood pressure.
- Sit with your arm extended and supported on a flat surface so that the upper arm is at the level of your heart.
- Keep your feet flat on the floor.
- Make sure the middle of the cuff is placed directly over the brachial artery (located just above the crease in your elbow) or, if taking a wrist measurement, over the radial artery (located on the wrist at the base of the thumb).
- Take two to three readings, one minute apart, and record the values on your Blood Pressure Progress Chart. If you prefer to track your numbers online, go to the American Heart Association's website, www.heart360.org.

of your blood pressure over time. Since there are no noticeable symptoms of high blood pressure, measuring it over time is the only way to measure your progress.

It has been shown that people who measure and track their

blood pressure themselves have superior results when it comes to getting their blood pressure under control. See the sidebar "Home Blood Pressure Measurement Instructions" on page 29 for the best results in measuring your blood pressure at home.

Choosing the Right Home Blood Pressure Monitor

You can purchase a home blood pressure machine at your local pharmacy, at a medical supply store, or online. The American Heart Association (AHA) recommends that you use a digital blood pressure machine that measures blood pressure at the upper arm, which is far more accurate than measuring at the wrist or the finger. Before you shop for a home blood pressure monitor, be sure to follow these simple tips: (1) Measure your upper arm and choose a monitor with the correct size cuff. (You can try the cuff on first and make sure it fits.) (2) Make sure the display shows your blood pressure values in a large, clear, easy-to-read display. (3) Check to see if your health insurance provider will cover the cost of a home blood pressure monitor. Many do. (4) Make sure that your blood pressure machine has been recommended by the dabl Educational Trust website, www.dableducational.org/sphygmomanometersdevices_2_sbpm.html#ArmTable. This ensures that the machine has been tested, validated, and approved. (5) Once you have purchased a device, ask your doctor to check it for accuracy against his or her office device.

You now understand the real danger of uncontrolled blood pressure, what the numbers mean, and how to measure and track your blood pressure numbers. In the next chapter, let's take a look at what drove your blood pressure up in the first place.

2

High Blood Pressure:
The Silent Killer

Ignorance more frequently begets confidence than does knowledge: it is those who know little, not those who know much, who so positively assert that this or that problem will never be solved by science.

—Charles Darwin

My patients routinely relay to me their doctor's concern over their blood pressure numbers. Despite their own anxiety, many tell me they are reluctant to take medications to control it, because they fear the notorious side effects. Let me make this as clear as possible: high blood pressure is an insidious disease that slowly eats away at your organs, ultimately cutting your life span. *It must be controlled*—with lifestyle first, and then with drugs, if necessary. In this chapter, I'll take you on a tour deep within your body to help you understand what kind of damage can occur after years of uncontrolled blood pressure. Sad to say, because high blood pressure is symptomless, many don't treat the disease until it's too late and the damage has already been done. Fortunately, with the lifestyle changes outlined in this book (and medications if prescribed by your physician), you can control your high blood pressure and reduce your risk of catastrophic complications.

THE NUTS AND BOLTS OF HIGH BLOOD PRESSURE

As you already know, blood pressure is the measure of the force against the walls of the arteries as the heart pumps blood through the body. High blood pressure is chronic excessive force on the arteries. There are several factors that determine your blood pressure. They include your heart rate (the higher the heart rate, the higher the blood pressure), the volume of blood in your vessels (the greater the blood volume, the higher the pressure), the amount of resistance in your blood vessels (the greater the resistance, the higher the blood pressure), and the thickness or viscosity of the blood (the thicker the blood, the higher the pressure).

Your heart is a muscular pump that normally beats between sixty and ninety times a minute. With each beat, your heart muscle contracts and propels freshly oxygenated blood into pipes that snake their way throughout the extensive winding network of blood vessels that permeate every square inch of the body (Figure 2.1). The arteries are a little like plumbing, but instead of being made of a hard, immovable substance, the "pipes" are a flexible, highly elastic

WARNING: HIGH-PRESSURE ZONE

Ever wonder why health professionals draw blood from veins and not arteries? It's because of the location and the dramatic difference in pressure. Veins are closer to the surface of the skin, so they are easier to locate with a needle and contain very little pressure. Arteries, on the other hand, are high-pressure zones. If your doctor or nurse were to draw blood from an artery, it would send a stream of blood squirting across the room with every heartbeat. If a major artery is severed, the high pressure can cause someone to bleed to death in minutes if left untreated. The closer to the heart the artery is, the higher the pressure and the faster the bleed—although a compromised artery anywhere in the body can be a life-threatening event.

organ made up of living cells. Keep in mind that the living nature of the arteries makes them fragile and highly susceptible to damage.

The purpose of the cardiovascular system is to transport oxygen and nutrients to every cell in the body and bring waste products away from the cells. The blood's journey begins as it is ejected with great force out of the heart and into the grand aorta, the largest

The Blood Vessel System

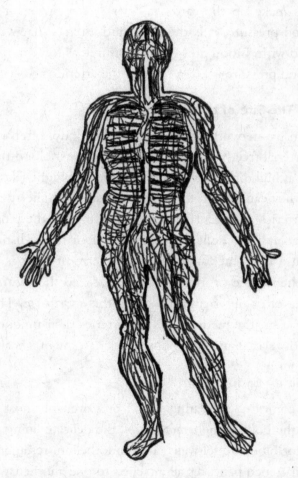

Figure 2.1 Each day approximately 2,000 gallons of blood circulate many times through about 60,000 miles of blood vessels that branch out and link to all the cells of our organs and body parts.

artery in the body. The blood continues on through progressively smaller arteries until it arrives at the smallest arteries, called *capillaries*, which are just one cell layer thick. This is the "exchange area," where oxygen and nutrients are dropped off to cells and waste products are picked up. The deoxygenated blood then continues its course through the veins—the return highways back to the heart and lungs—to dispose of the waste.

It is important to keep in mind that while the heart, arteries, and veins make up the cardiovascular system, when it comes to high blood pressure, it is the heart and arteries that we are most concerned with. Blood pressure is measured as force in the arteries. High blood pressure is *excess* force in the arteries.

Arteries: The Site of the Damage

The extensive network of arteries in your body, often referred to as the "arterial tree," is constructed to transport blood throughout the body at high pressure. Healthy arteries are highly elastic, meaning that they can stretch to handle occasional higher-than-normal forces. Arteries are circular in cross section, like the pipes in your house, yet unlike a solid pipe, they contain three distinct layers, each with a different function. The innermost layer is called the *intima*, the middle or muscular layer is called the *media*, and the external layer or outer casing is called the *adventitia*. The middle, muscular layer, the media, gives the arteries their unique ability to contract or relax. Figure 2.2 shows the anatomy of a healthy artery.

The Almighty Endothelium

When it comes to regulating blood pressure, the most important organ in the body is the *endothelium*, the delicate lining of cells on the interior blood vessel walls. The endothelium resembles a single sheet of flattened pancakes all attached to one another, with microscopic junctions between "pancakes," or cells. This layer is adjacent to the flow of blood and serves as a barrier between the blood and the inner layer of the arterial pipes, the intima. A healthy endothelium

Inside a Healthy Artery

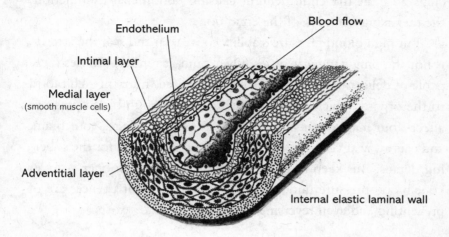

Figure 2.2   A cross-sectional view of a normal, healthy artery. Arteries consist of three layers: the intima, the media, and the adventitia. Coating the innermost layer, the intima, is a layer of smooth, flat endothelial cells collectively referred to as the endothelium. A healthy artery is flexible, elastic, and strong.

has three crucial characteristics: (1) it produces and secretes chemicals that keep the arteries relaxed and dilated, (2) the tight junctions between its cells block entry of anything abnormal from the blood into the intimal layer, and (3) its surface is slick and smooth and does not generate chemicals or molecules that let immune system cells or platelets (blood clotting cells) stick to its surface.

A dysfunction of endothelial lining cells is one of the root causes of hypertension, so those cells are a prominent player in the plan to control blood pressure. In future chapters you will learn how the Blood Pressure Down plan can heal the arteries and specifically the fragile endothelium.

WHY HIGH BLOOD PRESSURE IS SO DANGEROUS

High blood pressure, or excessive arterial force, can quietly damage your body before symptoms develop. If left untreated, the disease damages the body's lifelines, the arteries. High blood pressure also chips away at the endothelium, causing endothelial dysfunction, the menacing hallmark of the condition.

But high blood pressure's ability to weaken and scar the arteries is not the only danger it poses. Over time, it renders arteries incapable of delivering enough freshly oxygenated, nutrient-rich blood to the organs, which leads to tissue damage. High blood pressure affects four main organs: it strains your heart, damages your brain, and eats away at your eyes and your kidneys. Read on for the sobering details. But keep in mind the good news: the sooner you get your blood pressure under control, the better your chances are of preventing and even reversing damage if it already exists.

GOOD NEWS FOR A HIGH-PRESSURE NATION

Currently, the majority of adult Americans have abnormally elevated blood pressure. This is clearly a health catastrophe, as 50 percent of all new cases of coronary heart disease (our nation's leading cause of death) are attributed directly to high blood pressure. The good news is that if you control your pressure, you can cut your risk of dying from a heart attack by 20 percent, reverse organ damage, and significantly cut your risk of death from heart attacks and stroke, even if you have already been diagnosed with cardiovascular disease.

Sources: Wijeysundera HC, Machado M, Farahati F, et al. Association of temporal trends in risk factors and treatment uptake with coronary heart disease mortality 1994–2005. *JAMA* 2010;303:1841–1847; Cowan BR, Young AA, Anderson C, et al. Left ventricular mass and volume with telmisartan, ramipril, or combination in patients with previous atherosclerotic events or with diabetes mellitus. *Am J Cardiol* 2009;104:1484–1489; Verdecchia P, Sleight P, Mancia G, et al. Effects of telmisartan, ramipril, and their combination on left ventricular hypertrophy in individuals at high vascular risk. *Circulation* 2009;120:1380–1389.

WOUNDING THE ARTERIES

A healthy artery is flexible and strong, allowing blood to flow freely through the network (Figure 2.2). The endothelium is smooth and free of plaque buildup. Untreated high blood pressure creates chronic excess force that injures the delicate arteries, leaving them stretched, scarred, and prone to plaque buildup and blood clots. Damage to the inner layer results in inflammation and launches a cascade of events that promotes both arteriosclerosis (pronounced "ahr-teer-e-o-skluh-RO-sis"), or hardening of the arteries, and atherosclerosis (pronounced "ath-ur-o-skluh-RO-sis"), or plaque buildup within the arteries. This can block or lessen blood flow to many areas of the body, which can permanently damage your heart, brain, eyes, and kidneys. The higher the pressure, the greater the

---

EXCESS RESISTANCE: THE REAL PROBLEM

Most people with high blood pressure have a problem deep down within the arteries themselves, a relentless tightening of the vessels that results in high peripheral vascular resistance (PVR). There are four factors contributing to this excess resistance: (1) an intensification in the activity of the sympathetic nervous system (the part of the nervous system responsible for the fight-or-flight response); (2) a rise in the amount of calcium moving into the smooth muscle cells of arteries, constricting the cells and reducing the diameter of the vessels; (3) an upturn in oxidative stress and the production of harmful free radicals, leading to a dysfunctional endothelium; and (4) functional alterations in the structure of the arterial wall, such as thickening and hardening. All of the steps in the Blood Pressure Down plan target PVR in some form, easing the squeeze and helping you to get your blood pressure numbers to a healthier level.

Source: Blaustein MP, Leene FHH, Chen L, et al. How NaCL raises blood pressure: a new paradigm for the pathogenesis of salt-dependent hypertension. *Am J Physiol Heart Circ Physiol* 2012;302:H1031–H1049.

stress to the arteries and the faster the arteries harden and fill with plaque.

Another problem that can occur in the arteries is called an *aneurysm*. Chronic high pressure can overstretch the arteries and cause a section of the arterial wall to weaken. (Think of how constant force in an old garden hose can cause weak spots and stretching in areas of the hose.) An aneurysm occurs when the constant strain within the arteries exacerbates this weakening and causes one section of the artery to bulge. This can happen in any artery, but it is most common in the aorta, the largest artery in the body. If the aneurysm bursts, it can be a life-threatening event. Getting your blood pressure down will prevent and even reverse arterial damage that can lead to an aneurysm.

WOUNDING THE HEART

We've been talking a lot about arteries, but high blood pressure is also dangerous for your heart. The heart is a muscle, about the size of your fist, that functions as a pump to generate the pressure needed to move your blood along the miles of arteries in the body. There are four chambers in the heart: the left atrium, the right atrium, the left ventricle, and the right ventricle. The heart has its own special collection of arteries, the coronary arteries, which carry blood and nutrients such as oxygen to the heart muscle cells. Figure 2.3 shows the location of the major arteries that feed the heart.

Long-standing high blood pressure harms the heart in three ways: (1) it contributes to the process of plaque buildup (atherosclerosis) in the coronary arteries, which can result in a heart attack; (2) it can lead to an abnormal enlargement of the heart's left ventricle, a condition called *left ventricular hypertrophy*; and (3) it can result in complete heart failure. You should know that it is possible to reverse many of these malformations if the underlying problem

Danger Zones: Where Plaque Forms

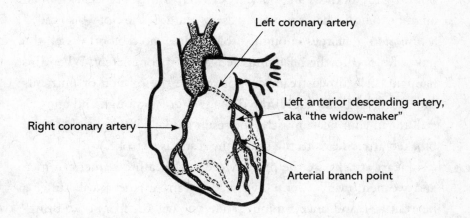

Figure 2.3   The major arteries that provide blood supply to the heart. Disease of the coronary arteries is the leading cause of death in the world. High blood pressure plays a major role in the development of heart disease.

of high blood pressure is treated in time. But if the condition has gone on for too long, the damage to the heart is usually permanent.

Atherosclerosis: The Making of a Heart Attack

A heart attack occurs when the blood supply flowing through the arteries that feed the heart (the coronary arteries) is cut off, resulting in damage to or death of part of the heart muscle. Blockage in the coronary artery is generally caused by a progressive disease process called *atherosclerosis*, severe arterial damage that results from years of plaque buildup in the artery walls. For decades, scientific studies have confirmed that high blood pressure fuels atherosclerosis. But how? Chronic high blood pressure continuously pounds away at the delicate lining of the inner arterial wall. This constant stress inflames the endothelium, making the wall more permeable to harmful cholesterol as well as allowing that cholesterol to accumulate. The hallmark of heart disease is the formation of small, volatile, cholesterol-filled plaque—precarious fatty deposits within the inner blood vessel wall. Eventually the plaque ruptures and is recognized by the body as an injury. Your body forms a blood clot in an attempt to heal what is perceived as a wound. If the clot—also called a *thrombus*—enlarges enough to block the whole blood vessel, the flow of blood to the heart muscle is cut off completely. When this happens, cells downstream do not receive the oxygen or nutrients they need, and they die. If the damage is great enough and enough cells die in your heart muscle, the result is a fatal heart attack. (If the blocked artery leads to the brain, the result is a stroke.)

Heart attacks are the primary cause of death of American men and women; every twenty-five seconds an American will suffer a heart attack, and once a minute someone will die from one. Bringing your blood pressure down is one of the best preventive actions that you can take to ensure that you don't get a heart attack.

Enlarged Left Ventricle: Badge of Disease

Uncontrolled pressure in the arteries places a relentless stress on the heart's pumping mechanism. Think of it this way: a garden hose that is narrowed requires that you open up the faucet some more to increase the water pressure. Extended periods of excess pressure in the arteries similarly increase the workload on your heart (the faucet). The left ventricle is the part of the heart that generates the power to propel the blood out of the heart and into the aorta and the miles of arteries that make up the arterial tree. When the resistance of the arterial tree is increased, the workhorse of the heart muscle—the left ventricle—is forced to pump harder. Over time, this causes the left ventricle to enlarge and stiffen, the condition called *left ventricle hypertrophy* (LVH). LVH can predispose you to a heart attack, heart failure, or sudden death.

Failing of the Heart

Eventually, persistent strain on the heart takes its toll, weakening the entire heart muscle and causing it to slowly wear out and

potentially fail to work entirely. This is called heart failure or con-
gestive heart failure: the inability of the heart to pump a sufficient
amount of blood to meet the needs of the body. Heart failure is
very common, affecting about 5.8 million Americans and killing
approximately 300,000 people every year.[1]

WOUNDING THE BRAIN

High blood pressure can severely weaken and damage blood vessels
that lead to the brain. Just like the heart, the brain has a network of
arteries that continuously feed brain tissue with freshly oxygenated
blood and nutrients. Persistent high blood pressure weakens the
walls of those arteries and can cause a thin spot to form. The weak
area fills with blood and balloons out, creating an aneurysm.

The potential effect of high blood pressure on the brain is
stroke, the third-leading cause of death in this country. There are

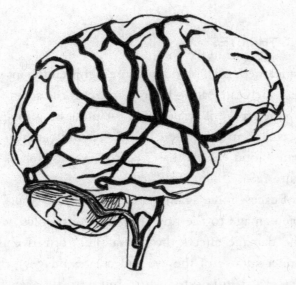

Figure 2.4   The major arteries that provide blood supply to the brain. High blood
pressure is the most important risk factor for developing a stroke.

two types of stroke: hemorrhagic and ischemic. Continuous high pressure can cause a "brain bleed," where the weakened artery wall breaks and blood leaks out, depriving part of the brain of oxygen and nutrients and causing brain cells to die. This is called a hemorrhagic stroke. About 13 percent of all strokes are hemorrhagic.

Another, more common kind of stroke is called an ischemic stroke. This happens when plaque ruptures and a blood clot forms, blocking blood flow. Again, brain cells die. About 87 percent of strokes are ischemic.

Since the brain is responsible for movement and thought, the death of brain tissue can result in slurred speech, memory loss, and muscle paralysis. The takeaway message is that high blood pressure is a powerful determinant of risk for both ischemic stroke and hemorrhagic stroke. The good news is that people with a normal blood pressure reading of 120/80 mm Hg have approximately half the lifetime risk of stroke compared to people with high blood pressure. Getting your blood pressure down will significantly reduce your risk of stroke.

WOUNDING THE EYES

As you just learned, high blood pressure significantly ups your odds of a stroke, which can lead to brain damage. If the area of the brain affected by the stroke is responsible for processing images, vision loss can occur. Untreated high blood pressure can also harm the tiny, delicate blood vessels that feed the eye, as well as the optic nerve (Figure 2.5).

Years of excess force against their fragile inner walls can cause microscopic damage to the tiny arteries, or arterioles, feeding the eyes. If the damage affects the retina (light-sensitive tissue that lines the inner surface of the eye and creates images), the disease is known as *hypertensive retinopathy*. Injury to the eyes from high blood pressure is cumulative, meaning that the longer your blood pressure is uncontrolled, the higher the likelihood of permanent

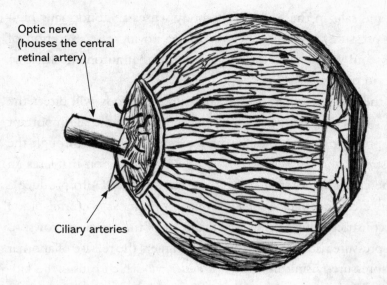

Optic nerve
(houses the central
retinal artery)

Ciliary arteries

Figure 2.5 The microscopic arteries that provide blood supply to the eye. High blood pressure can strain the blood vessels and the optic nerve, causing permanent vision problems.

vision damage. Getting your blood pressure down will significantly reduce your risk of going blind.

WOUNDING THE KIDNEYS

Chronic high blood pressure is extremely dangerous for your kidneys. *Hypertensive nephropathy* is the medical term for the damage to the kidneys that results from chronic high blood pressure.

First, a little background about these amazing organs. The kidneys have many vital functions in the body, all of which are required for maintaining good health. They cleanse the blood by filtering it, removing excess fluid and waste products, and then excreting the waste through the urine. The kidneys are sophisticated filtering machines. Tiny units called nephrons sift the blood; each kidney has about 1 million nephron units, each with its own arteriole—the small terminal twig of an artery.

What you may not know is that your kidneys and your blood pressure are inextricably linked. Kidneys regulate potassium level, acids, and salts in the body. If the body senses an abnormally high blood pressure, it will signal the kidneys to increase excretion of sodium and water—a feedback mechanism that automatically lowers blood pressure.

If the body senses too low a pressure, the body will direct the kidneys to increase production and excretion of the all-important blood pressure hormone called *renin*. Renin circulates through the bloodstream and triggers a complicated chain reaction that uses an enzyme called angiotensin-converting enzyme (ACE) to produce a substance called *angiotensin II*—your body's most powerful blood vessel constrictor. As a result, the diameter of the vessels narrows, so blood pressure rises. This scenario also triggers the release of another blood-pressure-raising hormone, *aldosterone*, which causes the kid-

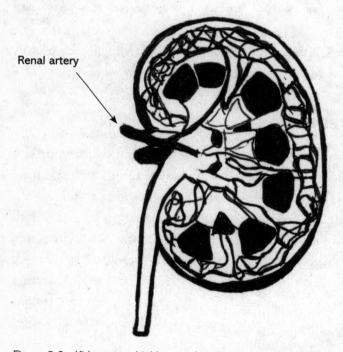

Renal artery

Figure 2.6 Kidneys are highly vascular organs, meaning they are packed with blood vessels. Kidneys are fed blood by both large-sized and small-sized arteries. High blood pressure is especially harmful to the smaller, highly fragile blood vessels feeding the individual nephron units. Damage causes a reduction in blood supply, resulting in disease.

neys to retain more water and sodium. The end result is an increase in blood pressure (as a result of blood vessel constriction and sodium and water retention). Some blood-pressure-lowering drugs work through the kidneys: ACE inhibitors lower blood pressure by blocking the production of angiotensin II, while diuretics lower blood pressure by increasing the kidneys' excretion of sodium and water.

Kidneys have a dense network of blood vessels and normally receive a high volume of blood flow. Just like in the rest of the body, chronic high blood pressure can wreak havoc on the walls of arteries in the kidneys, causing them to weaken and narrow in size or harden. As a result, blood flow is reduced, and the nephrons do not receive an adequate supply of nutrients. This shortage of blood makes it more difficult for the kidneys to perform their vital tasks. Eventually, dangerous levels of toxic wastes and fluid accumulate in the blood, a condition known as *uremia*. When this happens, the patient requires dialysis—a machine that performs the kidneys' blood-cleansing tasks. The eventual outcome is kidney failure, which is exactly what it sounds like: damaged kidneys that fail entirely to function. This condition requires regular dialysis or a kidney transplant, or else the patient will die. High blood pressure is the second leading cause of kidney failure (after diabetes).

SEXUAL DYSFUNCTION

Uncontrolled high blood pressure can result in sexual dysfunction in both men and women. In men, it damages the arteries that supply the penis, causing the arteries to harden (arteriosclerosis) or narrow (atherosclerosis). This reduces blood flow and hinders the ability to have and maintain an erection; the condition is called *erectile dysfunction*. In women, high blood pressure can damage the arteries leading to the vagina. Reduced blood flow to the vagina can result in decreased sexual desire, decreased ability to have an orgasm, and vaginal dryness.

High blood pressure can also cause an aneurysm in the renal artery, the main artery leading to the kidneys. As you already know, aneurysms can burst, resulting in life-threatening internal bleeding. Getting your blood pressure down will significantly reduce your risk of kidney disease, help preserve the kidneys' function, and protect your life.

RISK FACTORS FOR DEVELOPING HIGH BLOOD PRESSURE

Clearly, high blood pressure is a dangerous disease. So how did you get it in the first place? High blood pressure is an extremely complex disease that results from the interplay between environmental and genetic factors. While the exact set of causes differs widely from person to person, and some of them are out of your control, there are a multitude of factors that you *can* control. The Blood Pressure Down plan will ultimately tackle all of the changeable factors that predispose you to this disorder.

Family history. If your parents or siblings have high blood pressure, the odds are mighty good that you will develop it as well. Scientists have identified more than fifty genes that are associated with blood pressure irregularities. That said, you can't blame it all on your genes. Lifestyle changes can prevent and even reverse high blood pressure.

Age. Getting older is a risk factor; hence the old saying that your pressure should be 100 plus your age. As we age, at least in the West, our arteries stiffen, which as you have learned means a higher risk for elevated blood pressure. Our kidneys also become less functional with age, making it more difficult for the body to regulate salt. This raises blood volume and triggers a further rise in pressure. It's important to know that a rise in blood pressure with age is not a natural occurrence. There are isolated populations on the planet that demonstrate that this phenomenon is not inevitable.

Race. Your race affects your risk. African Americans are four times more likely than Caucasians to develop high blood pressure. Blood pressure problems are also more severe and develop earlier in blacks. This is largely because the African American population has higher rates of obesity and diabetes, two diseases that are related to the development of high blood pressure. Furthermore, scientists have discovered a gene, highly prevalent in blacks, that makes individuals much more susceptible to the blood-pressure-raising effect of salt. According to the American Heart Association, in salt-sensitive people as little as an extra half teaspoon of salt per day can raise blood pressure by as much as five mm Hg, whereas in non-salt-sensitive people, this amount of salt would have no effect on pressure.

Weight. Obese people are five times more likely to have high blood pressure than normal-weight individuals. Researchers have found that extra body fat activates two of the factors underlying elevated pressure we discussed in Chapter One: an overactive sympathetic nervous system and an overactive renin system. Lose body fat and your blood pressure will go down.

Kidney function. Too much renin is another risk factor for developing high blood pressure. When the kidneys produce too much renin, the result is twofold: (1) sodium retention in the blood, which leads to excess fluid volume, and (2) constriction of blood vessels, via the production of the highly potent vasoconstrictor called angiotensin II. Both scenarios raise blood pressure. This kind of high blood pressure is called *high-renin hypertension* or *renin-dependent hypertension*. Two-thirds of middle-aged Caucasian adults with high blood pressure have this type. People whose kidneys produce too much renin respond well to therapy with an ACE inhibitor, a type of drug that interferes with the actions of renin.

Other people have a type of high blood pressure called *low-renin hypertension*, a situation in which the elevated blood pressure is due not to high renin levels but more likely to other factors such as salt sensitivity. One-third of all people with high blood pressure have this type. Low-renin high blood pressure is more common in older adults, African Americans, and those with resistant hypertension. People with this type of hypertension often respond better to diuretic medications than to drugs that treat the consequences of elevated renin (such as ACE inhibitors). Your doctor can do a blood test to determine if you are a low-renin or a high-renin hypertensive.[2]

The Blood Pressure Down plan will help you fight abnormal kidney function and dilate your blood vessels, easing the pressure.

Metabolic syndrome. Metabolic syndrome is a combination of medical disorders that, when occurring together, predispose an individual to diabetes and heart disease. These disorders include high blood pressure, abdominal obesity, high triglycerides, low HDL, and insulin resistance. What is insulin resistance? In healthy people, the hormone insulin regulates the amount of sugar in the bloodstream and raises the activity of the parasympathetic nervous system, which relaxes and dilates blood vessels. In individuals with metabolic syndrome, the body resists the effects of insulin—the hormone cannot do its job. Instead the sympathetic nervous system overrides the blood vessel dilation that should occur, narrowing the arteries and resulting in an increase in blood pressure. The Blood Pressure Down plan will help you to lose weight (especially the dangerous belly fat characteristic of metabolic syndrome) as well as make your muscles much more insulin sensitive. And the exercises here will tame your sympathetic nervous system overdrive.

Unhealthy diet and sedentary lifestyle. A poor diet, especially one too high in bad fats and salty, high-calorie processed foods, will contribute to weight gain, create a mineral imbalance in the body, and raise your blood pressure. Not getting enough exercise also contributes to high blood pressure.

Cigarette smoking. It is a well-known fact that cigarette smoking increases risk for heart disease, but you may not know that this deadly habit also increases risk for developing high blood pressure. Work with your doctor to quit this toxic, life-shortening habit.

Low vitamin D. Vitamin D is the new hot vitamin in nutrition these days. Research is mounting showing a link between vitamin D deficiency and high blood pressure. When there is not enough vitamin D circulating in the blood, the kidneys try to compensate by releasing copious amounts of renin, resulting in salt retention, increased blood volume, blood vessel constriction, and, ultimately, high blood pressure.

Diet, Not Drugs, Should Be the First Line of Defense

You now understand the basics of blood pressure mechanics and the importance of controlling and keeping your blood pressure down. Untreated high blood pressure can put you in an early grave: more than 800,000 Americans die each year from blood-pressure-related diseases. The good news is that high blood pressure is a disease that is highly treatable, for a low cost. Get your blood pressure down and you will prevent medical complications and premature mortality.

You have learned that prescription drugs should not be the first line of defense against high pressure. A blood-pressure-lowering lifestyle is the safest, most effective, and ultimately the best medicine to fight this insidious disease. If you are already taking medication, lifestyle therapy can reduce the number of drugs you take and the dosage of your drugs, lessen the medication side effects, and certainly reduce the cost—all of which clearly emphasize the invaluable role of natural lifestyle therapy. Unfortunately, many patients and physicians fail to underscore the vital role lifestyle therapy plays in the prevention and treatment of high blood pressure.[3]

Now it's time to learn about the ten lifestyle steps in the Blood Pressure Down plan, which capitalize on the ability of certain foods—plus exercise—to reduce and stabilize blood pressure. These foods use a variety of mechanisms in your body to keep your heart healthy and prevent the development or recurrence of heart and blood vessel disease. Several of the dietary steps in the Blood Pressure Down plan work in a druglike fashion, almost the dietary equivalent of taking a diuretic (such as hydrochloro-thiazide), a calcium channel blocker (such as amlodipine), or an angiotensin receptor blocker (such as valsartan). Take this more natural lifestyle approach either alone or in combination with your physician-prescribed medications and watch your blood pressure plummet—without the side effects!

Blood Pressure Down: A Potent Natural Combination Therapy

Let food be thy medicine and medicine be thy food.

—Hippocrates

Reducing your blood pressure without drugs is easier than you think. The Blood Pressure Down plan is a combination approach of losing a little bit of weight, eating six types of foods, and exercising, developed from my extensive research on the best way to naturally reduce blood pressure. The plan works because it harnesses the specific blood-pressure-lowering potential of several simple diet and lifestyle manipulations. The combination of these is far more effective than a single food or exercise. Why? Each component has been scientifically proven to lower blood pressure to a different degree. Remember, with abnormal high blood pressure, every millimeter counts—for every 20 mm Hg increase in systolic blood pressure number above normal, there is an approximate doubling of risk for heart attack and stroke.[1] Each component of the plan tackles your high blood pressure from a different angle; together, this potent natural combination therapy can lower blood pressure as much as most single prescriptions. In the next section, you will learn about the therapeutic blood-pressure-lowering lifestyle strategies, then put them all into action simultaneously, providing you with the safest and most effective natural method to get your blood pressure down.

COMBINATION LIFESTYLE THERAPY FOR OPTIMAL BLOOD PRESSURE MANAGEMENT

Your Life Is in Your Lifestyle

Treatment for all types of high blood pressure is classified as either lifestyle or pharmacotherapy. This book is about *lifestyle therapy*, the specific nondrug, natural modifications known to be the cornerstone of treatment for high blood pressure. As you have learned, lifestyle therapy should always be used first and foremost to prevent and treat high blood pressure.[2] Read on to get a better picture of the lifestyle modifications that you will combine to attain and maintain lifelong blood pressure control.

What Is Combination Lifestyle Therapy?

Combination lifestyle therapy is a hybrid of diet and exercise modifications for lowering blood pressure. There are varying opinions on the best combination. The U.S. government,[3,4] the American Heart Association,[5] the Canadian government,[6] and the British Hypertension Society[7] each have their own guidelines, as you can see in Table 1 on pages 54–55. Each of the six modifiable lifestyle factors listed here has been proven to significantly reduce blood pressure. This might seem overwhelming, but don't worry! I just want you to see how much evidence there is for all of these lifestyle modifications. In my plan I've put them all together for you, to multiply the blood-pressure-lowering power of each one.

DIET WORKS AS WELL AS DRUGS IN
LOWERING BLOOD PRESSURE

Is a blood-pressure-lowering diet as powerful as a starting dose of a blood-pressure-lowering prescription drug? The answer is a resounding yes! In 1995 the National Heart, Lung, and Blood Institute (NHLBI) funded a landmark study named the Dietary Approaches to Stop Hypertension, or DASH trial, which found that what you eat (or don't eat) can profoundly affect your blood pressure numbers. The DASH trial provided the first convincing scientific evidence that a nonpharmaceutical lifestyle treatment could significantly reduce blood pressure. The study illustrated that even when body weight and sodium intake were constant, dietary intervention alone significantly lowers both systolic and diastolic numbers by an average of 11.4 and 5.5 mm Hg in those with diagnosed high blood pressure and by 3.5 and 2.1 mm Hg in normal study participants. These drops are similar to those achieved by blood-pressure-lowering medication, showing that the simple daily combination of certain foods can be just as powerful as a blood pressure drug in getting your blood pressure down.

Sources: Sacks FM, Obarzanek E, Windhauser MM, et al., and the DASH Investigators. Rationale and design of the Dietary Approaches to Stop Hypertension trial (DASH): a multi-center controlled feeding study of dietary patterns to lower blood pressure. *Ann Epidemiol* 1995;5(2):108–118; Appel L, Moore TJ, Obarzanek E, et al., for the DASH Collaborative Research Group. A clinical trial of the effects of dietary patterns on blood pressure. *N Eng J Med* 1997;336:1117–1124.

Additional Scientific Support for the Efficacy of Natural Combination Therapy

Our strategy of piling on different lifestyle strategies to magnify the combined effect has been scientifically proven. For example, the ENCORE (Exercise and Nutrition Interventions for Cardiovascular Health) study tested the effects of three natural lifestyle therapies: nutrition, weight loss, and exercise.[8] The ENCORE study was

Table 1. A Comparison of Lifestyle Recommendations Proven to Effectively Lower Blood Pressure

Recommendation	JNC 7[3]	NHLBI[4]	AHA[5]	CHEP[6]	BHS[7]
Lose weight	Maintain normal body weight (BMI 18.5–24.9)	Maintain normal body weight for adults (BMI 18.5–24.9)	For overweight and obese individuals, lose weight, aiming for a BMI < 25; for nonoverweight individuals, maintain a desirable body weight	Maintain a healthy body weight (BMI 18.5–24.9) and waist circumference (smaller than 102 cm for men and smaller than 88 cm for women)	Maintain ideal body weight and a BMI of 20–25
Adopt a DASH-type dietary pattern	Consume a diet rich in fruits, vegetables, and low-fat dairy products, with a reduced content of saturated fat and total fat	Consume a diet rich in fruits, vegetables, and low-fat dairy products, with a reduced content of saturated and total fat (DASH eating plan)	Consume a diet rich in fruits, vegetables (8–10 servings per day), low-fat dairy products (2–3 servings per day), and reduced in saturated fat and cholesterol	Follow a diet that is reduced in saturated fat and cholesterol, one that emphasizes fruits, vegetables, and low-fat dairy products, dietary and soluble fiber, whole grains, and protein from plant sources	Consume a diet rich in fruits, vegetables, and low-fat dairy products, with reduced content of saturated and total fat
Reduce sodium intake	Reduce dietary sodium intake to no more than 2.4 g/day	Reduce dietary sodium intake to no more than 2.4 g/day	Lower salt (sodium chloride) intake as much as possible, ideally to 1.5 g/day of sodium	Restrict dietary sodium to less than 2,300 mg/day (1,500 mg to 2,300 mg/day in hypertensive patients)	Reduce dietary sodium intake to < 2.4 g/day

Increase potassium intake	—	Maintain adequate intake of dietary potassium (> 3500 mg/d)	Increase potassium intake to 4.7 g/d, which is also the amount provided in DASH-type diets	—	—
Limit alcohol intake	Limit consumption to no more than 2 drinks per day (1 oz or 30 mL alcohol [e.g., 24 oz beer, 10 oz wine, or 3 oz 80-proof whiskey] in most men and no more than 1 drink per day in women and lighter-weight persons)	Limit alcohol consumption to no more than 1 oz (30 mL) alcohol (e.g., 24 oz beer, 10 oz wine, or 2 oz 100-proof whiskey) per day in most men and to no more than 0.5 oz alcohol per day in women and lighter-weight persons	For those who drink, consume ≤ 2 alcoholic drinks per day (men) and ≤ 1 alcoholic drink per day (women)	Limit alcohol consumption to no more than 14 units per week in men or 9 units per week in women	Men ≤ 21 units per week; women ≤ 14 units per week alcohol (in the UK, a unit of alcohol is defined as 10 mL, about 8 g)
Engage in regular aerobic exercise	Regular aerobic physical activity such as brisk walking (at least 30 minutes per day, most days of the week)	Engage in regular aerobic physical activity, such as brisk walking, at least 30 minutes per day, most days of the week	—	Perform 30 to 60 minutes of aerobic exercise 4 to 7 days per week	Engage in regular aerobic physical activity, such as brisk walking, for at least 30 minutes most days

a randomized clinical trial (RCT), the gold standard of scientific research or experiment, which randomly places subjects by chance into study groups. The RCT is one of the simplest and most powerful tools in clinical research, because it allows for establishing a cause-and-effect relationship between the intervention and the outcome. In the ENCORE RCT, 144 overweight and obese unmedicated people with prehypertension or stage 1 high blood pressure were randomly assigned to one of three groups for a period of four months: the DASH diet alone, DASH combined with a weight management program (a weekly cognitive-behavioral therapy session plus a program of walking, jogging, or biking for thirty minutes three times a week), or a control group (instructed to follow their usual eating and exercise routine).

The main outcome was a significant reduction of blood pressure in all groups, but the combination treatment was clearly the most powerful. The control group lowered their blood pressure by 3.4 mm Hg (systolic) and 3.8 mm Hg (diastolic), and the DASH diet alone group lowered blood pressure by 11.2 mm Hg (systolic) and 7.5 mm Hg (diastolic). By comparison, the combination group following the DASH diet plus weight loss lowered their blood pressure by a whopping 16.1 mm Hg (systolic) and 9.9 mm Hg (diastolic); their average weight loss was five pounds per month. Why the control group showed a small but significant drop in pressure despite no intervention is not clear. It may have been indicative of a placebo effect or their "usual" diet and exercise habits. What is crystal clear from this landmark study, however, is the value of combining exercise, weight loss, and diet to reduce blood pressure. Weight loss, exercise and a DASH diet produced an additional 5/2 mm Hg drop in pressure beyond the DASH diet alone!

Another RCT divided fifty-one sedentary overweight middle-aged men into two groups. One followed their usual diet; the other followed a reduced calorie diet.[9] Each group was then further subdivided into a program of either light exercise (stretching and cycling against zero resistance) or vigorous exercise (high-intensity cycling three times a week). After four months, the dieters lost an average of twenty-one pounds. Only the dieters exhibited a significant reduction in blood pressure, an average of 8.5 mm Hg systolic and 6.0 mm Hg diastolic. And the vigorous exercise dieters showed an even greater reduction in blood pressure than their lighter-exercise counterparts. The conclusion from the study was that the synergy of diet plus higher-intensity exercise (thirty minutes three times per week) is far more effective in reducing blood pressure than either on its own.

Reducing Blood Pressure and Cutting Prescription Drug Use in the Elderly

Getting on in age and worried about your escalating blood pressure and the side effects of all that medication? Then you will be interested to learn about the TONE (Trial of Nonpharmacologic Interventions in the Elderly) study, which analyzed the synergistic effect of losing weight and cutting sodium in almost one thousand people ages sixty to eighty who had high blood pressure and were taking a single prescription drug to treat it.[10] Study participants were randomized to one of three lifestyle interventions (sodium reduction, weight loss, or a combination of both) or to a control group (no intervention). The sodium groups reduced their sodium intake to less than 1,800 mg/day, and the weight loss subjects were asked to achieve and maintain at least a ten-pound weight loss. The results? When compared to the control group, over twenty-nine months the sodium-reduction group lowered their need for antihypertensive medications by 31 percent, the weight loss group by 36 percent, and the combination by a whopping *53 percent*!

Interestingly, the combined group was the most successful in keeping their blood pressure under control after discontinuing medication. The study's author concluded that a combination of healthy lifestyle changes can help elderly Americans become less dependent on antihypertensive medication.

The Big Guns for Fighting Blood Pressure: Millimeter by Millimeter

As you can see, there's no shortage of proof that natural combination therapy works. The prestigious groups of doctors and scientists of the government's JNC 7 committee have outlined approximately how many millimeters each of the top lifestyle therapies lowers systolic blood pressure (the top number):[11]

1. **Losing weight** can lower blood pressure up to 20 millimeters
2. **Adopting a DASH-style diet rich in fruits, vegetables, and low-fat dairy** can lower blood pressure up to 14 millimeters
3. **Cutting dietary sodium to less than 2,400 mg/day** can lower blood pressure up to 8 millimeters
4. **Exercising thirty minutes a day, most days of the week,** can lower blood pressure up to 9 millimeters
5. **Limiting alcohol consumption to one drink a day for women and two for men** can lower blood pressure up to 4 millimeters

You can be sure that each of these well-established strategies is included in the Blood Pressure Down plan—along with several additional less well-known but equally effective lifestyle steps. Used together, these strategies form a lifestyle "attack" on different systems related to blood pressure regulation, with a much greater impact than any single therapy.

THE BLOOD PRESSURE DOWN PLAN

You now know that high blood pressure is usually silent but always treacherous and that you must get it down. If you are not ready to get on the prescription bandwagon—or if you want to get

DANGER: KIDS WITH HIGH BLOOD PRESSURE

High blood pressure is not just an adult disease. Sad to say, more and more children and adolescents are being diagnosed. This may be because of the childhood obesity crisis. A recent study followed more than eleven hundred children, averaging ten years of age, for five years. Researchers found that overweight kids were three times more likely to develop high blood pressure. It may be unimaginable to think that children could get heart attacks or strokes, but these are very real side effects of high blood pressure. Getting our kids exercising and eating healthfully will help them lose weight and lower their blood pressure, as well as help reduce the epidemic of type 2 diabetes—improving their health now and helping them become healthier adults.

Source: Eckert GJ, DiMeglio LA, Yu Z, Jung J, Pratt JH. Intensified effect of adiposity on blood pressure in overweight and obese children. *Hypertens* 2011;58:818–824.

off—you can rest assured that the combination of natural, safe, and highly effective lifestyle methods outlined in these pages will get your blood pressure under control. Blood Pressure Down takes six individual blood-pressure-lowering foods—all scientifically shown to independently reduce blood pressure—and combines them on a daily basis with a manageable amount of weight loss, salt restriction, exercise, and relaxation. Combining all these proven blood-pressure-lowering strategies is as effective as combining several types of blood-pressure-lowering drugs. All the ingredients are available at your local supermarket and are no more dangerous, exotic, or expensive than bananas, yogurt, or walking.

Each step in the plan lowers your blood pressure several millimeters in a slightly different way, so the combination approach is substantially stronger than a single therapeutic treatment. Going on the "mineral diet" I prescribe (high amounts of potassium, magnesium, and calcium-rich foods), for example, lowers pressure by balancing the electrolytes in your bloodstream. Getting in daily aerobic exercise such as brisk walking, on the other hand, lowers pressure by boosting internal production of nitric oxide, a natural substance that acts like Valium for endothelial cells, relaxing and widening the arteries. A daily dose of both the minerals and exercise cuts pressure much more than either in isolation. In this way, all ten steps of the Blood Pressure Down plan work together to pack a very powerful punch in lowering blood pressure.

Ready to Bring Your Blood Pressure Down?

The next ten chapters provide a set of simple, healthful food and exercise prescriptions that give safe and measurable blood-pressure-lowering results in as little as four weeks. If you're at high risk of developing high blood pressure or already have the disease, these ten lifestyle changes can literally save your life. Think of all ten steps as the equivalent of a daily prescription pill—it's essential to do your best to get them all in. You'll keep track of your progress using the Ten-Step Daily Checklist located in Appendix 2, the same tool my patients use. Read on to begin with Step 1 of the daily checklist and start now to get your blood pressure down!

Part II

The Ten-Step Blood Pressure Down Plan

4

Step 1: Lose Five Pounds

℞ Eat Fewer Calories and Burn More

SMALL WEIGHT LOSS, BIG BLOOD PRESSURE REWARD

You can do this! Aim for losing just five pounds this next month (that's just a touch over one pound a week) and you will be taking the most powerful lifestyle step toward getting your blood pressure down. According to the World Health Organization, high blood pressure is often caused by being overweight combined with physical inactivity.[1] In fact, as many as 50 percent of overweight men and women who have high blood pressure developed the disease *because* they are overweight.[2] Armed with this knowledge, you can now take action and lose that weight for good. Many of my patients feel daunted by the task of losing weight, but take heart—even a modest weight loss results in a very significant fall in blood pressure.

How Much Should You Weigh?

Scientists screen for weight categories that may lead to health problems using a measurement called *body mass index* (BMI). Your BMI is a number calculated from your weight and your height, and it is a reliable indicator of body fat for most people. (You can easily calculate your BMI yourself by using the equation in Appendix 3.) A BMI above 25 strongly predisposes you to developing high blood pressure. But never fear—if your BMI tops 25, losing just 5 percent of your body weight can help slash your blood pressure levels for good.

WEIGHT LOSS NORMALIZES BLOOD PRESSURE

Weight gain increases blood pressure, and weight loss reduces it—it's as simple as that.[3] You learned in Chapter Three that of all the lifestyle modifications scientifically proven to reduce blood pressure, weight loss is the most effective. According to the JNC 7 report, a mere five-pound weight loss can reduce blood pressure by up to 5 mm Hg, and a ten-pound weight loss can yield a whopping 10 mm Hg drop.[4] (That's the blood-pressure-lowering equivalent of cutting out a full teaspoon of salt a day *and* exercising five days a week!)

What If You Are Not Overweight?

High blood pressure is more common in people who are overweight, and as noted, losing weight has its advantages in minimizing high blood pressure in overweight individuals. However, if you are at a healthy body weight (have a BMI between 18.5 and 25) and your pressure is high or you have a strong family history of hypertension, then losing weight will not be advantageous for you, so it's best to focus on the other nine lifestyle steps to get your blood pressure down. But that's not to say that you will not benefit from the healthful eating principles outlined in this chapter, so I encourage you to read on!

Healthy Lifestyle, Healthy Arteries

What's good for the waistline is also good for the arteries, according to researchers at Harvard Medical School.[5] The famed Nurses' Health Study II, begun in 1989, followed more than 116,000

GOT HARD-TO-TREAT HYPERTENSION?
LOSE THE WEIGHT, GET OFF THE DRUGS

An exciting study at the University of Mississippi Medical Center found that adding a lifestyle weight loss program to the regimen of older people with hard-to-treat blood pressure (stage 2) works miracles. More than one hundred elderly overweight men and women with uncontrolled high blood pressure were placed in one of two groups: a weight loss group or a control group. After approximately two years, the weight loss group had, not surprisingly, lost weight. But they had also reduced both the number of drugs and the dosage of blood pressure medication required to control stage 2 high blood pressure.

Source: Jones DW, Miller ME, Wofford MR, et al. The effect of weight loss intervention on antihypertensive medication requirements in the Hypertension Optimal Treatment (HOT) study. *Am J Hypertens* 1999;12:1175–1180.

women nurses, ages twenty-five to forty-two, from states all around the nation. Every two years for almost two decades, the nurses filled out questionnaires about their diets and health. In 1991, a section of the original group comprising over 80,000 healthy young women with normal blood pressure at the start of the study was followed until 2005. During that fourteen-year period, 12,319 cases of new hypertension were reported. When researchers analyzed the data, they found that the nurses with the lowest blood pressure were the ones who routinely had incorporated six healthy lifestyle factors into their lives.

So what are these six secret blood pressure relaxers? The first—and the one with the most impact on whether or not women developed high blood pressure—is maintaining a healthy body weight. (In this study, a healthy weight was defined as a BMI under 25.) The five additional factors were: daily vigorous exercise of thirty minutes on average, a high score on following the DASH diet (more on this diet in a few chapters), modest alcohol intake, limiting use of non-narcotic analgesics (such as Tylenol) to once a week or less, and intake of a daily folic acid supplement. (Note that four of these six steps are part of the Blood Pressure Down plan.)

So how much of an effect did these six lifestyle factors have on the nurses' blood pressure? The study showed that when practiced in combination, this six-part lifestyle "cocktail" reduced the risk of high blood pressure by an incredible *80 percent*! (Body weight alone was the most powerful predictor, which will not come as a surprise to you.) The authors concluded that a combination of life-style factors has the potential to prevent the majority of new-onset cases of high blood pressure in young women.[6]

You Are What You Don't Eat

A more recent study combined data from three huge long-term studies of thousands of men and women, and clearly showed the relationship between what you eat and what you weigh.[7] Here the subjects (nurses, doctors, dentists, and veterinarians) were again required to complete detailed health questionnaires every two years, and were followed for a period of twelve to twenty years. Interestingly, those people who gained the most weight over the years had similar eating habits. The greatest contributors to weight gain were (in descending order) french fries, potato chips, sugar-sweetened drinks, red and processed meats, other forms of potatoes, sweets and desserts, refined grains, other fried foods, 100 percent fruit juice, and butter. As you read on, you'll notice that, with the exception of potatoes (which are OK when cooked without added saturated fat), none of these foods is included in the Blood Pressure Down eating plan. Also not surprising was the find-ing that those who gained the least weight ate a diet heavy in fruits, vegetables, and whole grains. Exercise also played a role in keeping the weight off—those who had the most regular physical activity gained 1.76 fewer pounds over each four-year period than their less active counterparts.

CUT OUT THE LIQUID SUGAR: LOSE WEIGHT AND MILLIMETERS

You might know that soda and other sugar-sweetened beverages such as fruit drinks are the most commonly consumed beverages in the United States—and the leading source of added sugars in our diets. What you may *not* know is that scientists have linked higher blood pressure to people who consume more glucose and fructose. Both are sweeteners found in high-fructose corn syrup, the most common sweetener used by the beverage industry. The good news? Studies have shown that if you cut out the sugary drinks from your day, you will lose weight *and* lower those millimeters in one fell swoop!

Sources: Brown I, et al. Sugar-sweetened beverage, sugar intake of individuals, and their blood pressure: International Study of Macro/Micronutrients and Blood Pressure. *Hypertens* 2011;57:695–701; Chen L, Caballero B, Mitchell DC, et al. Reducing consumption of sugar-sweetened beverages is associated with reduced blood pressure: a prospective study among United States adults. *Circulation* 2010;121:2398–2406.

Super Science Supports the Power of Weight Loss and Blood Pressure Reduction

Based on data from scores of scientific studies, it is clear that losing a few pounds has a dramatic effect on blood pressure. Let's take a look at two meta-analyses, a sophisticated statistical technique in which the results of numerous studies are analyzed all together. In these cases, the meta-analyses took data from randomized clinical trials to explore the efficacy of weight loss for both preventing and treating high blood pressure.[8,9]

The first meta-analysis reviewed sixteen well-designed studies to determine the impact of weight loss on long-term blood pressure control ("long-term" was defined as at least two years). Results showed that for adults with a starting BMI of 35 or less, an eleven-pound weight loss would result, on average, in a 5.6 mm Hg reduction in systolic blood pressure.[10]

The second meta-analysis examining the effect of weight reduction on blood pressure was published in 2003 in the journal *Hypertension* and evaluated twenty-five randomized controlled clinical trials. Of the nearly five thousand participants, half had been diagnosed with high blood pressure and approximately one-fourth were taking antihypertensive medication. The results showed that weight loss of just two pounds was associated with an approximate 1 mm Hg reduction in both systolic and diastolic blood pressure. (Larger blood pressure reductions were observed in populations taking antihypertensive medications.) The loud and clear takeaway message? Lifestyle modifications that promote weight loss should be a major component in treating and preventing high blood pressure.[11] (The general rule of thumb is that a one-pound weight loss will result in an approximate 1 millimeter reduction in blood pressure. That means if you are overweight and lose twenty pounds, you can reduce your blood pressure by a phenomenal 20 mm Hg!)

Got Prehypertension? Weight Loss Works!

The Trials of Hypertension Prevention (TOHP) was a long-term, large-scale study conducted during the 1990s to assess the feasibility and efficacy of seven nonpharmacological interventions in the prevention of high blood pressure among two thousand men and women with prehypertension, or readings at the high end of the normal range. (The seven interventions were: weight loss, sodium reduction, stress management, and nutritional supplements of calcium, magnesium, potassium, and fish oil.)[12]

After six months, only two of the seven intervention groups exhibited a significant reduction in blood pressure: the weight loss group and the sodium restriction group. The participants in the weight loss group lost an average of about thirteen pounds with a corresponding blood pressure reduction of 3.8/2.5 mm Hg—a far greater drop than that observed in the sodium restriction group. The researchers concluded that weight reduction was the most effective of the seven strategies for lowering blood pressure. This study adds to the growing body of evidence that losing just a few pounds is incredibly powerful in getting that blood pressure down if you have prehypertension.

LOWER BLOOD PRESSURE = LONGER LIFE

Here's a dramatic statistic: people with high blood pressure who were able to get it down with drugs and lifestyle showed a gain in life expectancy of about *twenty years* compared to untreated middle-aged people. That was the finding of a huge randomized, controlled clinical trial of almost five thousand patients with high blood pressure, published recently in the prestigious *New England Journal of Medicine*. According to the researchers, each month of high blood pressure therapy was associated with a one-day prolongation of life expectancy.

Source: Kostis JB, Cabrera JC, Cheng JQ, et al. Association between chlorthalidone treatment of systolic hypertension and long-term survival. *JAMA* 2011;306(23):2588–2593.

WEIGHT LOSS 101

The Blood Pressure Down plan sets a doable goal for almost anyone: just five pounds in four weeks, a small but significant weight loss that will teach you the fundamentals of losing weight safely and permanently. Health professionals recommend a weight loss of no more than one to two pounds per week. This is the rate of weight loss that targets body fat—the blood-pressure-raising pounds that you want to lose.

Now that you know that losing just a few pounds works like a charm to lower those millimeters of mercury, how do you actually go about this oftentimes difficult task? Diet fads come and go, but sensible weight loss techniques stand the test of time. Losing weight and keeping it off requires you to make changes in *what* you eat, changes in the *way* you eat, and changes in your daily movement routine. As tough as losing weight can be, one small step at a time makes it possible.

Despite what you may have heard, calories *do* count when it comes to losing weight. That's why we're going to take a back-to-basics approach of counting calories. The fact is that to lose one pound of body fat a week, you need to eat 500 fewer calories a day. You can accomplish this by eating 250 calories less than you normally eat and burning the additional 250 calories with exercise. What is the most painless way to eat fewer calories? The answer, in

WHAT'S ON THE MENU? EXCESS SALT AND CALORIES!

We love restaurants! More than 80 percent of us go out to eat at least once a week. Hot off the presses, a new nutritional analysis of nearly 31,000 menu items from 245 of America's top chain restaurants has bad news for those of us interested in watching our weight and controlling our blood pressure. A whopping 96 percent of restaurant entrees fell outside the USDA's recommendations for healthy amounts of saturated fat and sodium. Sodium was particularly problematic, with the average entrée packing in over 1,500 mg—more than you should eat in an entire day! Appetizers fared even worse in the salt and calories department, with an average of 2,023 mg of sodium and 813 calories (and that's just the appetizer). Keep in mind that the calories add up quickly: the average entrée clocks in at 674 calories; side dish, 260; salad, almost 500 calories; specialty beverage, 418; and dessert, 429. Clearly, if your goal is to take in less than 1,500 mg of sodium and a maximum of 2,000 calories in a day, a single restaurant meal can easily put you over the top.

Source: Wu HW, Sturm R. What's on the menu? A review of the energy and nutritional content of US chain restaurant menus. *Public Health Nutr* 2012. DOI:10.1017/S136898001200122X.

one word, is substitution: substitute healthful low-calorie foods for the high-calorie or high-fat foods that you typically eat.

How Much Should You Eat?

For the sake of simplicity, and to jump-start your weight loss, the Blood Pressure Down plan provides a two-week meal plan containing approximately 2,000 calories per day. Since women usually have a smaller stature than men, they need fewer calories. According to the Dietary Guidelines for Americans, adult women generally require 1,800 to 2,400 calories, and adult men usually need somewhere between 2,000 and 3,000 calories, depending on their activity level. I suggest that if you are a woman (or a man of smaller stature), cut out about 200 calories a day from the sample meal plans. I also provide two meal breakdown patterns that offer guidelines about how to divide up your daily calories between various meals and snacks; women can use the 1,800-calorie pattern, whereas men can use the 2,000-calorie pattern. (For a more individualized meal plan, you can use an online calculator to estimate the number of calories you need to eat to lose weight safely, such as the one available at www .caloriescount.com. Then use a calorie-count book to adjust your meal plan accordingly.) Use the Ten-Step Daily Checklist in Appendix 2 to ensure that you are eating a range of necessary food groups and partaking in a healthful, balanced eating plan.

1,800-Calorie Meal Breakdown (women or smaller-stature men)

Breakfast	300 calories
Snack	100 calories
Lunch	400 calories
Snack	100 calories
Dinner	600 calories
Extras	300 calories

2,000-Calorie Meal Breakdown (most men)

Breakfast	300 calories
Snack	100 calories
Lunch	500 calories
Snack	100 calories
Dinner	700 calories
Extras	300 calories

You will build your meals with as many of the blood-pressure-lowering foods outlined in Chapters Three through Eight as possible. The two weeks of sample meal plans for the 2,000-calorie version, located in Appendix 7, give you sample breakfast, lunch, dinner, and snack ideas incorporating the six foods and food groups outlined in Chapters Six through Eleven. The meal plans have done all the calculations for you.

In the future, for keeping track of calorie counts in the foods you choose to eat, I recommend that you utilize a good online site; there are many, such as www.nutritiondata.com. I also recommend that you purchase a good calorie-count handbook as well as a restaurant guide. Two of my favorites, which include calorie and sodium content, are *The Calorie King Calorie, Fat, and Carbohydrate Counter 2012* by Allan Borushek, RD (Family Health Publications), and *Dr. Jo's Eat Out Healthy* by Joanne V. Lichten, PhD, RD (Nutritfit Publishing, 2012).

Take Ten to Lose Five

You are on your way to losing just a few pounds, which will guarantee you a healthful drop in blood pressure. Before you begin to shed those pounds, keep in mind these ten important tips for losing weight and keeping it off:

1. **Lose weight at a safe rate.** When it comes to losing weight and keeping it off, slow and steady wins the race. Weight lost too quickly often returns—and sometimes brings unwanted additional pounds. The safest diets promote weight loss of no more than two pounds (or 1 percent of total body weight) a week, which reduces the risk of health problems associated with more rapid weight loss (more than three pounds per week).[13]

2. **Calorie control is the secret to weight control.** Research has proven time and again that when it comes to weight loss, the old principle holds true: eat fewer calories than your body expends and you will lose weight, regardless of the percentage of carbohydrates, fat, and protein in the diet.[14] That's not to say that some food groups aren't better at facilitating weight loss than others. The type of food you select can boost your metabolism and help you stay fuller and satisfied longer. Protein, for example, reduces appetite and costs your body the most calories to metabolize.[15] Fiber is filling, and high-fiber foods tend to be more healthful, making them ideal snacks for keeping your hunger at bay. Fill up on "free foods"—fresh fruits and veggies—at meals and snacks. You can eat unlimited servings of these. Yes, unlimited! Nobody ever gained weight from eating too many apples or carrots.

3. **Keep track of your eating and exercise.** Numerous studies have found that people are most successful at losing weight and maintaining healthy habits when they record the type and quantity of food consumed.[16] To help you accomplish your weight loss and blood pressure goals, be sure to keep track of your food intake and exercise output on the Ten-Step Daily Checklist in Appendix 2.

ELECTRONIC WEIGHT LOSS

I urge all of you to perform one simple daily task that has proven time and again to help people stay on track and follow a healthy lifestyle: the simple act of keeping a food and exercise diary. It doesn't have to be anything fancy; just the act of writing down what you eat does the trick.

If you are like me and love free stuff, then you might like to take advantage of the myriad free online weight management sites that allow you to track your food and exercise routines. Here is a rundown of three excellent sites.

1. **SparkPeople.** This is one of the most popular sites around (12 million users and growing). It offers tons of stuff such as food and exercise tracking as well as weight tracking and social networking.
2. **FitDay.** Another wildly popular free food and exercise tracking site (over 6 million strong).
3. **MyPlate.** Livestrong.com's MyPlate allows you to set weight loss goals and track exercise and food intake. It has one of the largest online food libraries. Almost 4 million people belong to MyPlate.

If you are a smartphone or tablet user, you may prefer to track your diet and exercise habits using an app. Here are three of my favorite free apps for use on your portable devices:

1. **MyFitnessPal.** A huge social networking community, MyFitnessPal allows you to log food and exercise when you are out and about.
2. **LoseIt!** Another excellent free food and exercise diary used by millions of people. LoseIt! offers recipes, social networking, goals, and diet and exercise tracking.
3. **Daily Challenge.** This is not just for weight loss—it's a great tool to help you set any kind of small daily goals. It links to social media and is available as both a smartphone app and a Web application.

4. **Weigh yourself once a week.** Frequent weighing helps you lose weight and keep it off; not weighing yourself is associated with greater weight regain.[17] Set a time, place, and day of the week when you can record your weight (using approximately the same weight of clothing and without shoes). Keep track of your weight on the Body Weight Graph in Appendix 2.

5. **Portion size does count.** We live in a supersize society where bigger is perceived as better. The fact is, over the past forty years portion sizes in convenience foods and at restaurants have gotten larger, contributing to the ever-expanding American waistline. Some food items have more than doubled in size, adding additional calories to your plate and unwanted pounds to your body. When it comes to packing on the pounds, this may just be the biggest problem. Imagine that you're going back in time, shrinking the food on your plate and the number on the scale! Try eating from smaller plates—it tricks your mind into thinking you ate more than you really did.

6. **Cut down on certain foods, or cut them out completely.** If you want to learn to live leaner, calorie-rich foods must either be omitted entirely or savored in small amounts. Deep-fried foods, for example, contain at least double the number of calories as the same food baked or broiled. Animal protein contains high-quality protein but also tends to come packaged with lots of saturated fat and cholesterol—ingredients that bump up the calorie count considerably (as well as clog up the arteries). Opt for lean vegetable protein (beans, lentils, soy, and nuts) as often as possible. If you do want animal protein, choose only grilled, roasted, or broiled, and opt for seafood or skinless poultry for a fraction of the calories of fatty red meats.

FOOD FOCUS: CUT IT OUT OR ADD IT IN TO LOSE WEIGHT

In one study that followed nearly five hundred overweight and obese postmenopausal women for four years, researchers analyzed the eating behaviors most conducive to both short- and long-term weight loss. Over the short term (six months) the following behaviors were shown to be utilized by the successful weight losers:

- Cut it out: desserts, eating out often, sugar-sweetened beverages (such as soda, teas, and juices), fried foods
- Add it in: fish

At forty-eight months the following eating behaviors were associated with the greatest long-term weight loss:

- Cut it out: desserts, sugar-sweetened beverages, fried foods, and also meats and cheeses
- Add it in: fruits and vegetables

You can see from the results of this study that making a few simple changes in your eating habits can clearly help you to lose those excess blood-pressure-raising pounds!

Source: Gibbs BB, Kinzel LS, Gabriel KP, et al. Short- and long-term eating habit modification predicts weight change in overweight postmenopausal women: results of the WOMAN study. *J Acad Nutr Diet* 2012;112:1347–1355.

7. **Drink a lot of calorie-free fluids.** The large majority of the liquids you drink should be calorie-free. Water is perfect, and unsweetened tea and sparkling water are also great choices. A common dictum among nutritionists is "Never drink your calories; chew them!" Make sure to clear out all the sugary drinks from your refrigerator and pantry. If you don't have them available, you won't drink them.

8. **Eat small, frequent meals.** Study after study has shown that eating smaller, more frequent meals is the best approach to losing weight. When you eat, your body burns calories to digest the food. Eating at least five times per day (like the three meals and two snacks on the Blood Pressure Down plan) allows you to burn extra calories during the digestive process multiple times per day. Eating frequently also helps to control your hunger level, keep your blood sugar on an even keel, and decrease food cravings. When you are ravenous, you are less likely to make healthy choices.

9. **Substitute, substitute, substitute.** No question about it—eating less is hard to do. One of the best techniques you can utilize to prevent feelings of deprivation is to substitute tasty lower-calorie alternatives for higher-calorie, less healthful foods. Don't think so much about what you shouldn't eat; instead focus on what you can eat *more* of.

10. **Combine diet and exercise for better health, fitness, and weight control.** The most successful programs for promoting health and long-term weight control combine exercise and diet.[18] Balancing daily exercise with a calorie-controlled, nutritious eating plan is the best prescription for promoting health, fitness, and weight control.

HOW LOSING WEIGHT LOWERS BLOOD PRESSURE

Scientists are still figuring out how losing pounds works to tackle your blood pressure numbers. There are a couple of different hypotheses.

Method of attack #1: The most important benefit of losing weight is that it curtails the overactivity of the sympathetic nervous system. This mediates your body's fight-or-flight response for a calming, blood-pressure-lowering effect on the blood vessels.

SUBSTITUTIONS MAKE LOSING WEIGHT EASIER

Try these simple swaps:

- Egg substitutes or egg whites for whole eggs
- Nonstick spray for oils and butter
- Grilled and roasted meat and veggies for fried
- Sauces and salad dressing on the side
- Salsa instead of creamy, buttery sauces
- Nonfat dairy (fat-free milk, yogurt, sour cream) instead of low- or full-fat
- Baked potatoes and roasted fries for french fries
- Sparkling water or unsweetened iced tea for soda
- Water-packed tuna rather than oil-packed
- Fresh fruit, homemade desserts, or dark chocolate for fatty baked goods
- One glass of red wine instead of sugary cocktails

(Certain drugs work the same way. For example, beta-blockers such as metoprolol block the connection of the chemicals epinephrine and norepinephrine with their beta receptors, blunting the sympathetic nervous system.)

Method of attack #2: Excess body fat taxes the heart and blood vessels. Why? Fat cells are an active type of tissue that requires an extensive network of blood vessels to deliver oxygen and nutrients and remove waste products. In fact, it has been estimated that one pound of body fat contains about a mile of blood vessels.[19] Shedding just a small amount of body fat will reduce the body's demands on your circulatory system, thereby lowering blood pressure. Extra body fat places a heavy burden on the heart, too—it has to pump extra blood as well as counteract excess resistance within the blood vessels. Weight loss eases the load of the heart and reduces vascular resistance. No need to aim for unrealistic weight loss—losing just a few pounds is enough to yield a sizable, stable drop in blood pressure.[20] Don't let the perfect be the enemy of the good!

As you can see, losing just a few pounds can make a colossal dent in your blood pressure numbers. In the coming chapters, I'll walk you through the specific foods to eat—and avoid—but for now, the most important thing to remember is to create that daily calorie deficit. Control your portions, eat lighter, and exercise more, and you will be taking one of the most effective lifestyle medicines available for getting your blood pressure down! In the next chapter you will learn about the second-most-effective nondrug therapy for taming your numbers and see how the simple act of limiting your intake of the most toxic blood pressure mineral there is—ubiquitous in our food supply—can make your numbers plummet.

5

Step 2: Cut the Salt

℞ Eat a Maximum of 1,500 mg of Sodium Every Day

Our food supply is tainted. The fact is that salt, America's prized condiment, is actually a slow poison. Excess sodium intake is inextricably linked to the development of serious diseases in American women and men, namely, heart disease (the number one killer) and stroke (the number three killer). In fact, a whopping 90 percent of us will eventually develop high blood pressure from a lifetime of too much salt. As you have learned, high blood pressure predisposes you to heart attacks, stroke, kidney disease, and blindness. But oh, how we Americans love our salt! A new report from the Centers for Disease Control and Prevention states that nine in ten U.S. adults eat an unhealthy level of sodium every day.[1] The good news is, cut the salt and you will slash your blood pressure numbers. Let's see why this is so.

THE SALT OF THE EARTH

What Is the Difference Between Salt and Sodium?

The words *salt* and *sodium* are sometimes used interchangeably because most of the sodium we eat is in the form of salt. Think of salt (sodium chloride) as the transport vehicle for the mineral sodium. All forms of common salt contain 40 percent sodium and 60 percent chloride by weight.

While too much salt is dangerous, we also need it—both sodium and chloride are vital minerals that we *must* eat. Our cells need them to stay healthy, and our bodies can't make them.

SALT AND SODIUM CHEAT SHEET

Salt to sodium: To convert grams (g) of salt to milligrams (mg) of sodium, divide the salt figure in grams by 2.5 and then multiply by 1,000. So (grams of salt ÷ 2.5) × 1,000 = milligrams of sodium.

Sodium to salt: To convert milligrams of sodium to grams of salt, multiply the sodium figure in milligrams by 2.5 and then divide by 1,000. So (milligrams of sodium × 2.5) ÷ 1,000 = grams of salt.

Salt is such a vital nutrient that it has seeped through human history. Wars have been fought over it, empires created and destroyed by it. It was even once a form of legal tender (Roman soldiers were paid in salt; the word *salary* is derived from the Latin word for "salt.") Because salt can be used for food preservation, it enabled agricultural growth prior to refrigeration.

The differences among the various types of salt you see in the supermarket lie in the size of the grains and the additives they contain. Keep in mind that the mineral sodium is responsible for raising blood pressure—sodium is the health culprit in salt. Although salt is a major contributor of sodium to our diets, you should be aware that sodium in other forms is also a component of many products in the supermarket.

There are many reasons the processed food industry has doused its products with salt. Salt increases shelf life, and it's a cheap preservative. Plus the taste of salt is learned and it is addictive. People become habituated to high concentrations of salt in their food, which increases demand for salty products. For meat processors, a higher salt content increases the weight of the product at no cost to the producer (salt has a high water-binding capacity). Moreover, salty foods increase thirst, which helps sales of soft drinks and alcoholic beverages.[2] It's no wonder that salt manufacturers, the soft drink industry, and several types of food manufacturers have banded together to perpetrate the idea that salt is not involved in promoting high blood pressure.[3]

How Much Is Too Much?

While our bodies do need salt to survive, in modern times salt consumption has rocketed to exorbitant amounts—and we are seeing the adverse health effects. Since the 1970s, salt intake has risen by 69 percent in women and 48 percent in men.[4] According to the National Academy of Sciences, our bodies require just a tiny amount of sodium—500 milligrams a day, the quantity found in ¼ teaspoon of salt. And yet the average American consumes *eight times* this minimum amount.

THE SALT SITUATION: HOW MUCH ARE WE REALLY EATING?

Major health organizations recommend that our maximum daily intake of salt be 1,500 milligrams of sodium or 3.8 grams of salt per day. Most Americans easily consume almost three times that amount—or over 4,000 milligrams of sodium or 10 grams of salt, per day.

Why is this so? For starters, we use heaping amounts of salt as a seasoning. But it's also because outrageous amounts are hidden in processed and restaurant foods—foods we tend to overconsume. Your eating habits must change if you want your blood pressure to plummet. As you will soon learn, there are plenty of low-sodium foods on the supermarket shelf as well as seasoning alternatives that are tasty *and* healthy for the arteries.

Where Does Salt Come From?

Salt is obtained from the evaporation of seawater, or from the mining or drilling of underground salt deposits. Most of the salt we consume comes from the mining of huge salt deposits left in dried salt lakes throughout the world.

Salt from the Sea or the Earth: Beware of Both

The American Heart Association (AHA) asked a group of one thousand people nationwide whether they thought sea salt was a low-sodium alternative to salt.[5] Sixty-one percent believed this fallacy

---

SALT BY ANY OTHER NAME . . .

Salt is available in many forms, all with the same amount of sodium and chloride by weight. Each form of salt listed below contains a high percentage of the blood-pressure-raising villain sodium. So take all the health claims on these products with, well, a pinch of salt:

- Table salt: a fine-grained salt used for cooking and at the table.
- Kosher salt: a coarse-grained salt with no additives.
- Sea salt: contains other minerals; available in either fine-grained or coarse-grained forms. Produced by evaporation of seawater.
- Pickling salt: a fine-grained salt used for brines.
- Specialty salt, such as popcorn salt: a mixture of salt with other seasonings.
- Seasoned salt: a salt blend typically including herbs and other seasonings.

Source: International Food Information Council Foundation.

> ## WHAT ARE SALT SUBSTITUTES?
>
> Salt substitutes are salts in which some or all of the sodium has been replaced with another mineral, such as potassium or magnesium. In an effort to get that salty taste, we may tend to overconsume these substitutes; if they contain regular salt, this will provide you with too much sodium. And salt substitutes containing potassium chloride, if taken in excess, can be harmful if you have kidney problems or are taking medications that cause potassium retention.

was true. There's plenty of hoopla on the nation's radar concerning sea salt, marketed as a health food either alone or as an additive to a plethora of products erroneously thought of as "healthful." But the fact is, sea salt and table salt are almost identical, chemically speaking. The main difference between sea salt, kosher salt, and table salt is in the processing. Table salt has been mined from inland underground deposits, stripped of many of its natural minerals, and combined with an anti-caking ingredient, such as calcium silicate, to prevent clumping. Table salt also often has added iodine—an essential nutrient required for normal thyroid functioning.

The bottom line is that although your body needs some sodium to function properly, most people eat far too much sodium, which contributes heavily to high blood pressure. Cut out all forms of added salt used for seasoning (including table salt, sea salt, and kosher salt) and you will take a huge step in getting, and keeping, your blood pressure down.

Shaking Up the Guidelines?

The AHA recommends that most Americans strive to cap their sodium intake at 1,500 mg/day, or a little over ½ teaspoon of salt. But that's just a fraction of what the average American eats. Salt saturates the American food supply. While most authorities estimate average sodium consumption at 4,000 mg of sodium per day, a

NO MAN IS WORTH HIS SALT

The Yanomami Indians are a tribe of approximately twenty thousand people who live in villages in the Amazon forest on the border between Venezuela and Brazil. The Yanomami live a very active lifestyle without any added salt in their diet. Their average blood pressure is 95/61 mm Hg—making the Yanomami the people with the lowest recorded mean blood pressure on earth. (And their blood pressure does not increase with age.) By contrast, in the United States—where we eat an average of over 4,000 mg of sodium (10 grams of salt) daily—systolic blood pressure rises with age by an average of 7 mm Hg per decade after age thirty. That may not sound like a lot, but over the average life span that is the difference between 120 and 148 mm Hg. Moreover, a meta-analysis of twenty-eight randomized clinical trials involving nearly three thousand people from around the world found that cutting salt intake in half to less than 5 grams per day (for an average of four weeks) lowered blood pressure by an average of 5/3 mm Hg in hypertensives and 2/1 mm Hg in those with normal pressure.

Sources: Mancilha-Carvalho JJ, Souza e Silva NA. The Yanomami Indians in the INTER-SALT study. *Arq Bras Cardiol* 2003;80(3):295–300; He FJ, MacGregor GA, Singh GM, Danaei G, Pelizzari PM, et al. The age associations of blood pressure, cholesterol, and glucose: analysis of health examination surveys from international populations. *Circulation* 2012;125(18):2204–2211. He FJ, MacGregor GA. Effect of modest salt reduction on blood pressure: a meta-analysis of randomized trials. Implications for public health. *J Hum Hypertens* 2002;16:761–770.

more recent and alarming statistic estimates that the average man in the United States consumes 10.4 g of salt a day (the equivalent of 6,200 mg of sodium) and the average woman consumes 7.3 g a day (4,400 mg of sodium)[6]—nearly triple the maximum daily amount.[7]

WHERE'S THE SALT HIDING?

Where does all this sodium in our day come from? Even if you took away the salt shaker, you'd still be left with the lion's share of

SWIMMING IN SALT

Here are some salt statistics that you need to know:

1. **Nine in ten American adults eat too much salt every day.** If you are eating food from a box, a bag, a can, a bottle, or off a menu, odds are you are consuming excessive amounts of harmful sodium. The less processed your food, the less salt you'll eat. Stick to fresh, whole foods when possible and order simple, plain food at a restaurant.
2. **Almost half of the sodium we eat comes from only ten types of foods.** See the sidebar "Ten Salty Foods Americans Love to Eat" and do what you can to cut back.
3. **Cutting salt reduces health care costs.** Reducing the amount of sodium Americans eat by 1,200 mg a day (the amount in half a teaspoon of salt) could save up to $20 billion a year in medical costs. Cut the salt, save our health care system!

Sources: Centers for Disease Control and Prevention. Usual sodium intakes compared with current dietary guidelines—United States, 2005–2008. *Morbidity and Mortality Weekly Report* 2011. Oct21:1413–1417; Centers for Disease Control and Prevention. Where's the sodium? There's too much in many common foods. *CDC Vital Signs, February 2012.* www.cdc.gov/VitalSigns/Sodium/index.html.

sodium intake. This is because most of the sodium comes not from what we add to our food at home but what gets added in by others who cook or process our food. There are three important factors to understanding where the salt lurks in your day:

1. The *types* of food you consume matter (see the sidebar "Ten Salty Foods Americans Love to Eat").
2. *Who* prepares the food matters. Processed food is the number one source of salt, with 65 percent of that sodium coming from store-bought foods and 25 percent

coming from restaurant foods. Only about 10 percent comes from the salt shaker or what we add while cooking at home.

3. The *brand* of food matters. Different brands of the same type of food often vary widely in their sodium content.

Analyzing your own eating habits will help you strategize ways to get the salt out of your food. Remember the two key sources—store-bought processed food and restaurant food!

TEN SALTY FOODS AMERICANS LOVE TO EAT

Beware of relying too much on your taste buds. There are plenty of foods with unacceptable levels of sodium that do not necessarily taste salty. For example, a large shake at McDonald's contains almost double the amount of sodium as a large french fries! A recent report from the Centers for Disease Control and Prevention showed that there are ten kinds of food that account for 44 percent of all the sodium Americans eat each day. Note that the foods we typically think of as the saltiest—chips, pretzels, and other salty snacks—actually came in last!

1. **Breads and rolls.** Although each serving is not that high in sodium, we eat many servings of these grains per day, which add up to a lot of salt at the end of the day. Rx: buy low-sodium brands.
2. **Luncheon meat** such as deli ham or turkey. Rx: don't eat processed deli meat, or buy low-sodium brands.
3. **Pizza.** Both frozen and restaurant pizza are out of control with salt. Rx: eat just one small slice, and reduce your sodium intake for the rest of the day.
4. **Poultry.** Rx: eat more plant sources of protein, which are practically sodium-free.
5. **Soups.** Rx: avoid eating soups unless you make them yourself using alternative seasonings.

6. **Cheeseburgers and other sandwiches.** Rx: avoid eating sandwiches unless you make them at home using lower-sodium ingredients.

7. **Cheese.** Rx: avoid eating cheese unless you keep a careful eye on your sodium intake for the rest of the day.

8. **Pasta dishes.** Rx: cook pasta dishes at home with your own tomato sauce, seasoned with delicious herbs.

9. **Meat dishes such as meat loaf.** Rx: avoid meat dishes and opt for vegetable sources of protein.

10. **Snack foods such as potato chips, pretzels, and popcorn.** Rx: eat air-popped popcorn seasoned with an alternative seasoning.

Source: Centers for Disease Control and Prevention. Where's the sodium? There's too much in many common foods. *CDC Vital Signs, February 2012.* www.cdc.gov/VitalSigns/Sodium/index.html

Learning the Label Lingo

Sodium is often hidden in food products, so make sure you become a food label sleuth. Pay particular attention to processed foods. As you scrutinize the ingredients list, watch out for the trilogy of *s*-words: *salt, sodium,* and *soda.* Here are a few in particular to look out for:

Monosodium glutamate (MSG)

Baking powder

Sodium alginate

Sodium ascorbate

Sodium bicarbonate (baking soda)

Sodium benzoate

Sodium chloride

Sodium caseinate

Sodium citrate

Sodium hydroxide

Sodium nitrate

Sodium saccharin

Sodium stearoyl lactylate

Sodium sulfite

Disodium phosphate

Trisodium phosphate

In addition to scrutinizing the ingredients list, look for the terms "sodium free," "low sodium," and "reduced sodium" on the front of the label, and always check the Nutrition Facts panel for the amount of sodium per serving. (Keep in mind that you may be eating more than one serving.)

Some over-the-counter medications even have sodium. For example, one dose of the nonprescription antacid Bromo-Seltzer harbors a whopping 761 mg sodium. Other OTC painkillers do not contain sodium yet can also raise your pressure. These include acetaminophen (Tylenol) and nonsteroidal anti-inflammatories such as ibuprofen (Advil, Motrin), aspirin, and naproxen (Aleve and Midol Extended Relief). Be sure to ask your doctor.

THE SCIENCE OF SALT

Salt and Pressure Go Hand in Hand

The fact that salt raises blood pressure is not new knowledge. Nearly five thousand years ago, an ancient Chinese medical scholar wrote these words of wisdom: "Hence if too much salt is used for food, the pulse hardens."[8]

According to the Council on Science and Public Health, the prevalence of high blood pressure in our population, including the age-related rise in blood pressure that we experience, is directly related to sodium intake.[9] This concept—the more salt in the diet, the higher the pressure—was confirmed by the INTERSALT study, a large-scale study of more than ten thousand men and women (ages twenty to fifty-nine) from fifty-two populations around the world.[10] Scientists documented that people who routinely eat low amounts of sodium (less than 1,265 mg, or around half a teaspoon of salt, per day) have lower blood pressure and exhibit a blunted age-related rise in blood pressure with age. People with higher sodium intakes, on the other hand, have higher blood pressure, and most go on to develop high blood pressure as they get older. This phenomenon prevailed for both men and women and for younger and older people.

HOW DOES SALT RAISE BLOOD PRESSURE? SCIENTISTS WANT TO KNOW . . .

We know that too much salt in the diet is a major cause of high blood pressure—and the single most important controllable factor responsible for the rise in blood pressure with advancing age in our culture. But how does salt cause this effect in the body? A recent review article (an article that summarizes the current state of research on a given topic) has shed a great deal of light on the connection. Over time, a high level of sodium in the blood triggers the hypothalamus (a region of the brain) and the adrenal glands (which sit just over the kidneys) to release a potent hormone called ouabain. Ouabain is one of a trio of key blood-pressure-raising agents circulating in the blood (along with aldosterone and angiotensin II). Ouabain produces and maintains abnormally high blood pressure in two ways: (1) it increases the activity of the sympathetic nervous system, which, as we have seen, encourages the constriction of blood vessels, and (2) it fosters the entry of calcium into the smooth muscle cells of the arteries, which constricts the cells and tightens up the arteries.

Source: Blaustein MP, Leene FHH, Chen L, et al. How NaCL raises blood pressure: a new paradigm for the pathogenesis of salt-dependent hypertension. *Am J Physiol Heart Circ Physiol* 2012;301:H1031–H1049.

Lower Salt Intake = Lower Blood Pressure

The data are crystal clear: cut the salt and your pressure will drop. Myriad randomized controlled clinical trials (the most powerful scientific method for determining cause and effect) have demonstrated the benefits of sodium reduction for blood pressure control, in both people with normal blood pressure and people with previously diagnosed high blood pressure.[11,12,13,14] A meta-analysis published in the *Journal of Hypertension* was based on seventeen trials involving modest salt reduction in people with diagnosed high blood pressure, and eleven similar trials in people with normal pressure.[15] Salt intake was cut by an average of 5 g/day (2,000 mg of sodium), and resulted in an average drop in systolic blood pressure/diastolic

Drugs plus Salt Restriction Work Better than Drugs Alone

Are you taking drugs for your pressure, so you're not too worried about your salt intake? Well, think again. Eating less salt makes those blood pressure drugs much more effective in those who truly need them. Scientists recently tested a low-salt diet on twelve subjects who had resistant hypertension, meaning their blood pressure was still high despite taking an average of more than three different blood pressure drugs every day. Subjects were placed first on a high-sodium diet (5,750 mg/day) for seven days and then were switched over to a low-sodium diet (1,050 mg/day) for seven more days. (The two interventions were separated by a two-week washout period.) The results? Blood pressure dropped an average of 22/9 mm Hg during the low-salt phase. The researchers concluded that high salt intake contributes to resistant hypertension. The takeaway message: salt restriction enhances the blood-pressure-lowering effect of prescription drugs.

Source: Pimenta E, Gaddam KK, Oparil S, Aban I, Husain S, Dell'Italia LJ, Calhoun DA. Effects of dietary sodium reduction on blood pressure in subjects with resistant hypertension: results from a randomized trial. *Hypertens* 2009;54(3);475–481.

blood pressure of 4.96/2.73 mm Hg in people diagnosed with high blood pressure and 2.03/0.97 mm Hg in people with normal pressure. That's a huge payoff for a doable dietary change!

You should know that not everyone responds to salt reduction the same way. Researchers have discovered that blacks, middle-aged and older people, and individuals with chronic diseases such as diabetes, hypertension, and kidney disease tend to exhibit a greater response to dietary sodium restriction.[16] So if you fall into any of these categories, all the more reason for you to halt the salt.

What Would Happen If We Cut Our Salt Intake Just a Little?

As we've learned, an overwhelming body of scientific evidence links high salt intake to higher blood pressure and increased risk of heart attacks and stroke, yet dietary salt intake in the United States continues to rise. This disturbing situation made scientists wonder what the health benefits would be of a population-wide reduction of salt intake.

In a recent study published in the *New England Journal of Medicine*, researchers used a computer model to forecast the potentially achievable health benefits of reducing salt intake population-wide by up to 3 g/day (1,200 mg of sodium). What did they find? A little less salt could go a long way toward preventing disease. The scientists concluded that if all of us cut our salt intake by just half a teaspoon per day, there would be close to 100,000 fewer heart attacks each year, strokes would decrease by 32,000 to 66,000, and the number of total deaths from cardiovascular disease would drop by up to 92,000 annually.[17]

According to the study, these benefits would affect all segments of the population and could prevent heart disease and strokes as much as reductions in smoking, obesity, and cholesterol levels. It would also be more cost-effective than using medications to lower blood pressure. These findings are an emphatic call to action for the federal government to regulate salt concentrations in processed,

SAVING MONEY AND LIVES

In addition to saving a million lives, just how much money could we save if Americans reduced their salt intake by 10 percent? According to a study published in the prestigious *Annals of Internal Medicine*, a lot. Researchers calculated that the nation would save an astronomical $32 billion a year in health care costs by making this small dietary change.

Source: Smith-Spangler CM, Juuaola JL, Enns EA, Owens DK, Garber AM. Population strategies to decrease sodium intake and the burden of cardiovascular disease in the United States: a cost-effectiveness analysis. *Ann Intern Med* 2010;152(8):481–487.

prepared, and restaurant foods, and for the FDA to require warning labels on high-sodium foods.

SUPERMARKET SALT SHOCKERS

Just how much salt is lurking in your food? You will be amazed at the absolutely outrageous amounts of salt that permeate nearly every morsel. Salt is hidden in many foods that most people simply would never suspect. Here are twenty salt shockers to eliminate from your day:

1. **Canned vegetables.** Canned foods are one of the biggest culprits of hidden sodium. One cup of canned cream-style corn contains 730 mg of sodium. Rx: if you must buy canned, rinse the food or buy low-sodium products.
2. **Packaged deli meats.** Four ounces of extra-lean turkey ham contains 1,164 mg of sodium. Rx: roast a fresh (unseasoned) turkey and slice the meat yourself, or check the labels and buy the low-sodium varieties.
3. **Bottled spaghetti sauce.** A typical half-cup serving (not enough to even coat your pasta) contains about 600 mg

of sodium. Rx: buy low-sodium versions or dilute the bottled sauce with no-salt-added canned tomatoes or chopped fresh tomatoes and herbs—or better yet, make your own sauce.

4. **Marinades and flavoring sauces.** Most people know that soy sauce is ridiculously high in sodium, but other sauces such as teriyaki (1 tablespoon contains 690 mg of sodium) and barbeque sauce (¼ cup contains 509 mg of sodium) are also loaded with sodium. Rx: use balsamic vinegar, fresh fruit juice, extra-virgin olive oil, and herbs for flavoring.

5. **Nuts.** Nuts are heart-healthy, but certain salted varieties carry an excessive salt load. One ounce of Planters salted peanuts contains 190 mg of sodium. Rx: eat unsalted nuts.

6. **Condiments.** Seemingly innocent condiments often pack a wallop when it comes to hidden sodium. Two tablespoons of regular ketchup contain 380 mg of sodium; 2 tablespoons of mustard contain about 240 mg; 1 tablespoon of drained capers contains 255 mg; 2 tablespoons of relish contain 250 mg of sodium. Rx: try just a touch of honey mustard, which contains much less sodium than regular, or go for the low-sodium versions of these condiments.

7. **Canned tuna.** One 6-ounce can of water-packed white tuna, drained, contains 560 mg of sodium. Rx: give the tuna a quick rinse before eating, or buy a no-salt-added variety.

8. **Seasoned breadcrumbs.** A small serving (¼ cup) of these salty crumbs provides you with 795 mg of sodium. Rx: switch to plain crumbs, with 233 mg of sodium per ¼ cup.

9. **Cornmeal.** Who knew? A measly 1 cup of self-rising yellow cornmeal contains 1,860 mg of sodium. Rx: use plain yellow cornmeal at just 4 mg of sodium per cup. To use this in recipes where the leavening is important,

replace the baking soda (the source of all the sodium) with a sodium-free version available at health food stores.

10. **Chicken broth.** You may already know that most cans of soup contain massive amounts of sodium, but did you know that just 1 cup of canned chicken broth can contain up to 1,050 mg of sodium? Rx: switch to one of the many varieties of low-sodium broths.

11. **Microwave popcorn.** This low-calorie, high-fiber snack can easily put you over your daily sodium limit, with from 160 to 620 mgs of sodium per bag. Rx: buy only low-sodium varieties of microwave popcorn, or better yet, pop your own popcorn in a brown paper lunch bag or air popper and season with alternative seasonings.

12. **Ready-to-eat breakfast cereals.** Seemingly innocent and healthy, cereal can actually contain more sodium than you need at breakfast. One cup of Honey Nut Cheerios contains 269 mg; 1 cup of raisin bran contains 362 mg; one packet of instant maple and brown sugar oatmeal contains 253 mg. Rx: go for the least processed cereals, such as plain oatmeal cooked without salt (2 mg of sodium) or puffed wheat (0 mg).

13. **Bagels.** This popular bread product can contain upward of 700 mg of sodium for a large plain bagel. (In fact, most bread products contain excessive amounts of sodium.) Rx: instead of bagels, choose brands of whole-grain bread with "low sodium" on the label.

14. **Salad dressings.** Most commercially prepared salad dressings contain way too much salt. Just 2 tablespoons of zesty Italian dressing contain 510 mg of sodium. Rx: your best bet is to avoid bottled dressings and dress your salad with extra-virgin olive oil and balsamic vinegar or fresh lemon juice.

15. **Cottage cheese and full-fat cheeses.** Many cheeses contain outlandish amounts of sodium. Just a 4-ounce

serving of fat-free cottage cheese contains 380 mg; ¼ cup of crumbled feta cheese, 418 mg; and 1 ounce of Parmesan, 454 mg. Rx: go light on your use of cheeses.

16. **Onion soup mix.** A single packet of onion soup mix contains two days' worth of sodium: a whopping 3,132 mg! Rx: use alternative flavor sources, or use just a quarter of the packet.

17. **Fast-food sub sandwich.** Hungry at the deli counter? That 6-inch cold-cut sub will satisfy your hunger pangs, but it also contains more than your daily recommended total of sodium: 1,651 mg. Rx: opt for the salad bar instead at lunchtime—make sure your salad is dressed with balsamic vinegar and olive oil.

18. **Potato salad.** One cup of potato salad will put you back 1,323 mg of sodium. Rx: go for a plain baked potato instead.

19. **Baked beans.** One cup of franks and beans contains 1,100 mg of sodium. Rx: skip the canned baked beans and use the low-sodium canned bean varieties.

20. **Low-fat cheeses.** Low-fat may sound healthy—but when food manufacturers take out the fat, they add in more sodium. One single slice of low-fat American cheese, for example, has 300 mg of sodium. Rx: nix the cheese or use just a touch of strong cheeses (such as blue or Parmesan) for flavor.

WHY EXCESSIVE SODIUM IS TOXIC

A Salt Magnet

When you ingest sodium, it enters the bloodstream. Sodium is a charged particle, and the electrical charge attracts water. So sodium tends to pull fluid from the tissues into the arteries, raising blood volume. When the volume of blood increases, the heart must work harder to circulate it, and the pressure against the blood vessel walls increases. Continuous pressure taxes the circulatory system, narrowing the blood vessels. Through those narrowed vessels, less blood flows through to body tissues, which harms the cells. This is why the first-line drug of choice for lowering blood pressure is the relatively innocuous diuretic (water pill), which increases the amount of water (and sodium) excreted by the kidneys.

I ❤ NEW YORK

Salt is fast becoming the new trans fat! Policy makers are pressuring food manufacturers and restaurants to curb their sodium levels. New York City has once again taken the lead, with a goal of having its residents reduce salt intake by 25 percent in five years. It might sound like a lofty goal, but the fact is, most of us consume far too much salt, and it would be better for *all* of us to eat less. So take a bite of the big apple (1 mg of sodium) and cut your sodium intake by 25 percent.

You may have heard about the salt-sensitivity debate. Research suggests that there are some individuals who are more sensitive to salt than others, meaning that they are more likely than most to develop high blood pressure when exposed to high levels of sodium. That said, 90 percent of people in this country go on to develop high blood pressure at some point in their lives, and one of the principal causes is the excessive salt load in the food we eat. So in effect, we are *all* salt sensitive sooner or later and should *all* cut back on our salt intake.

FDA Fails to Regulate Salt and Protect Our Health

Unfortunately, salt has skirted federal regulation—which in effect means that our government has failed to protect our health. This is because salt falls under the classification of GRAS, or "generally recognized as safe." This term is applied to substances that have been deemed by the government as safe to eat, so they are exempt from customary food additive requirements. Hence there has been no limit set on the amount of salt that corporations can add to processed and restaurant foods. This lack of regulation has led to wild abuse on the part of food companies in terms of saturating the food supply with sodium—and placed a considerable disease burden on our country.

How can we solve this problem? Changing the classification of salt to a food additive would require that food companies prove the safety of the amounts used. The Center for Science in the Public Interest, a nonprofit, Washington, D.C.–based consumer advocacy group that focuses on nutrition and health, food safety, and alcohol policy, has for thirty years been urging the FDA to take salt out of the GRAS classification, to no avail. In 2005, the center petitioned the FDA to set maximum levels of salt, but to date no regulatory action has been taken. We are behind the curve compared to other countries such as Canada, the United Kingdom, Finland, Australia, and New Zealand. These countries have all initiated voluntary salt-lowering programs in collaboration with food companies, and have had considerable success in reducing the salt content of processed foods.

We could certainly learn a thing or two from Italy, a country that has taken many initiatives to reduce dietary salt intake, including an evaluation of current salt intake habits. The Working Group for Dietary Salt Reduction in Italy has collaborated with bakers' associations to gradually reduce the salt content of bread (a major source of sodium intake in Italy) and has mounted educational campaigns to increase the population's awareness of the salt problem.[18]

SCIENTIFIC EVIDENCE LINKS LOWER SALT INTAKE WITH BETTER HEALTH

How Does Restricting Salt Lower Blood Pressure and Prevent Disease?

Salt not only raises blood pressure but can harm the body in additional ways. New evidence is surfacing showing that salt has deleterious effects that go far beyond blood pressure. Whether along with or independent of high blood pressure, excess sodium harms your arteries, heart, bones, kidneys, blood, and even your stomach. Here's how cutting back on this hazardous condiment will help protect you.

Method of attack #1: As noted previously, sodium is a mineral that attracts fluid, increasing blood volume and blood pressure. Cut the salt and you will lose the water and your pressure will drop.

Method of attack #2: Too much salt stiffens, thickens, and narrows arteries, creating greater resistance, which increases pressure.[19,20] Cut the salt and you will remove much of this arterial irritant, calming and relaxing the arteries.

Method of attack #3: Excess salt intake worsens the damage that high blood pressure causes to the left chamber of the heart. Left ventricular hypertrophy (LVH) is an excessive thickening of the left ventricle, the chamber that pumps the blood throughout the body. LVH is a dangerous situation, as it is the primary cause of heart failure. Cutting back on salt has been shown to potentially reverse the muscle thickening characteristic of this life-threatening disorder.[21]

LESS SALT = LESS STROKE

A large majority of strokes are caused by high blood pressure. A new study, hot off the presses, found that for every 500 mg of sodium intake per day over the AHA's 1,500 mg/day limit, a person's risk of stroke increases by 17 percent! Researchers from both the University of Miami and New York's Columbia University Medical Center analyzed data from nearly three thousand participants in the Northern Manhattan Study over a ten-year period. Those people who ate more than 4,000 mg of sodium per day (about what the average American eats) had a 2.6-fold increase in stroke risk compared to those who ate less than 1,500 mg.

Sources: Gardener H, Rundek T, Wright CB, et al. Dietary sodium and risk of stroke in the Northern Manhattan Study. *Stroke* 2012;43(5):1200–1205; Cappuccio FP, Ji C. Less salt and less stroke: further support to action. *Stroke* 2012;43(5):1195–1196.

Method of attack #4: A high salt intake is harmful to the brain. Scientists have documented a direct effect between salt intake and risk of stroke—in other words, the amount of salt a person eats is directly related to the risk of stroke.[22] Cut the salt and you automatically decrease your risk of this debilitating and often lethal cardiovascular event.

Method of attack #5: Salt is also harmful to your body's blood clotting mechanism. Excessive amounts of salt in the diet increase the tendency for blood platelets to stick to the cells that line blood vessels, thereby increasing the ability of blood to clot—the last lethal step in a heart attack or stroke scenario.[23]

Method of attack #6: A high salt intake can severely affect the health of your stomach and your bones. There is a well-known association between excess salt intake and stomach cancer,[24] as well as between salt and the weakening of your bones (demineralization and osteoporosis).[25]

TEN SURPRISINGLY SIMPLE TIPS FOR CUTTING BACK ON YOUR INTAKE OF SALT

1. **Eat more fresh foods.** As long as our food supply is laden with salt, your best bet is to make your own food. Substitute fresh and whole unprocessed foods for processed foods whenever possible. The vast majority of natural, unprocessed fruits and vegetables contain only a minimal amount of sodium. At the supermarket, routinely buy fresh or frozen produce (with no added salt). Frequent salad bars and load up on unprocessed fruit and veggies.

2. **When you are buying packaged foods, read and use the information on the food labels to allow easy comparison between brands.** Always check the ingredient list for sodium, MSG, baking soda, and other sodium-containing compounds. You will be surprised at the tremendous differ-

ence between products in terms of sodium content. Only buy boxes, cans, and bags of food with the words "low sodium" or "sodium free" on the front. ("Low sodium" is defined as less than 140 mg and "high sodium" is more than 480 mg per serving.)

3. **Rinse canned foods, and dilute high-sodium foods.** Buy low-sodium beans and tuna and rinse in a strainer to drain off more of the salt. Cook pasta, cereals, and rice without added salt. Add salt-free beans, veggies, or grains (such as brown rice) to take-out, packaged, or frozen foods to dilute the sodium count.

4. **Throw out the seasoning packets**. Flavor rice or pasta yourself, and keep your intake of boxed foods or canned soups to a minimum. Watch condiments such as soy sauce, teriyaki sauce, ketchup, mustard, pickles, capers, and olives; use very little or omit them entirely from your diet. Use sprays, balsamic and other types of vinegar, and extra-virgin olive oil to flavor your food without the salt!

5. **Just say no to convenience foods.** Cut down on foods that come in a box, bag, or bottle (other than unsalted nuts or dried fruit). Pass on the take-out pizza—salty bread doused with salty tomato sauce and topped off with salty, fatty cheese. Remember, you can make almost anything from scratch, quickly, easily, and without spending hours in the kitchen. Think how you can use your rice cooker, Cuisinart, slow cooker, and blender to prepare foods. Salt-free seasoning blends, nuts and seeds, dried fruit, vinegars, and even peanut butter can be used for flavoring.

6. **Order it your way.** When eating out, order plain food without added sodium. Take care to customize your order, and ask for your food to be prepared without salt. Be sure to bring a copy of the Chef Card (see Appendix 5) with you to the restaurant to give to your waiter or directly to the chef. Order sauces and dressing on the side. Ask for condiments that are low in sodium. Watch the take-out or cheap eats—salt makes cheap food taste better.

7. **Use herbs and spices in lieu of salt.** Eat at home as often as possible, cooking fresh foods. Eliminate added salt and use chopped fresh herbs and spices to flavor food. Herbs such as rosemary, parsley, dill, chives, cilantro, and basil; spices such as cinnamon, cumin, and nutmeg; and seasonings such as lemon and lime juice, hot sauce, wasabi paste, vinegar, pepper, and salt-free seasoning blends all make great salt substitutes.

8. **Get rid of the salt shaker.** A dash of table salt contains about 155 mg of sodium, so be careful. Keep the pepper mill handy on the table, along with hot sauce and spice mixes. Find lower-sodium alternative seasonings that appeal to your taste buds. Be adventurous and flavor foods with sliced fresh ginger, garlic and garlic powder, a touch of horseradish (1 tablespoon of prepared horseradish contains 47 mg of sodium), and other lower-sodium condiments.

9. **Check medication ingredient labels.** Scrutinize the labels of all over-the-counter medications such as antacids for sodium content. Look for low-sodium varieties instead.

10. **Savor your salt.** Save those salty favorite foods for a special treat. Sodium in foods you consume frequently can really add up, so be sure to watch portion sizes of bread, and cut way back on (or eliminate) processed meats, deli meats, sodium-heavy cheeses, and restaurant and frozen pizzas and pasta dishes. When you do splurge on a salty treat, watch your sodium intake especially carefully for the rest of the day. Use higher-sodium condiments such as ketchup, barbeque sauce, mustard, pickles, olives, and Worcestershire sauce sparingly.

Beyond Blood Pressure: Salt's Destructive Effects

In summary, too much salt in your mouth not only is a major contributing factor to your blood pressure problem but also damages other bodily functions and organs, including:[26]

- Stiffening and narrowing of arteries, especially arteries feeding the heart, brain and kidneys
- Promotion of atherosclerosis (process of plaque buildup in the arteries, the root cause of heart attacks and stroke)
- Promotion of functional changes in the heart muscle that weaken it, such as left ventricular hypertrophy
- Increased tendency of blood to clot
- Additional harm to the kidneys (already wounded by excessive blood pressure), especially in people with kidney disease
- Harm to the skeletal system (weakened bones)
- Increased risk for stomach cancer
- Increased risk of dementia

Take control of your salt intake and you will be taking action to consume less sodium—the slow poison.

FILLING THE PRESCRIPTION

Eat no more than 1,500 mg of sodium every day. This can be done without sacrificing taste if you slowly but surely train your taste buds. Aim for eating at home more often, shop wisely and buy fresh whole foods more often, and flavor foods with healthful sodium-free ingredients.

Hold the Salt, Save Lives

I hope that you now realize the urgent need to reduce sodium consumption. There is simply too much salt in the foods we eat. We are a drive-through-window nation with an insatiable taste for cheap, salt-saturated processed food. Deemed "the forgotten killer," excess salt consumption clearly compromises health.[27] Sad to say, sodium is on our plates but apparently not on our minds—a recent survey found that 59 percent of us are "not concerned" about our dietary intake of this stealthy villain.[28] This is despite an overwhelming amount of irrefutable scientific evidence that too much sodium in the diet raises blood pressure, whereas restricting intake lowers it.

In light of these findings, it would appear prudent to answer the American Heart Association's call to action: the public, health professionals, the food industry, and the government must intensify efforts to reduce the sodium intake of all Americans to a reasonable level.[29] We must pressure our government to institute regulations for food manufacturers and restaurateurs, requiring them to reduce the salt content of our food.

Meanwhile, millions of Americans continue to succumb to disease caused or complicated by excess salt in our food supply. The Harvard School of Public Health found that of the 2.5 million deaths in the United States in 2005, 400,000 were directly attributed to high blood pressure. Among the dietary factors examined, high dietary salt intake had the largest effect, responsible for 4 percent of all adult deaths.[30]

In this chapter, you have learned that less salt translates into lower blood pressure and less disease. Take charge of your blood pressure, your health, and your life by standing up against salt overload in your own body and in our society. But blood pressure is far more than just sodium. Deficiencies in three complementary minerals are equally guilty in the promotion of high blood pressure. Consumption of certain quantities of these three key minerals has been scientifically proven to tame those millimeters, so load up on the minerals discussed in the next three chapters and you will be shocked at how quickly and safely you can get your numbers down.

6

Step 3: Eat Bananas

℞ Eat 4,700 mg of Potassium Every Day

OK, we've talked about what you need to cut out of your life—extra pounds from around your waistline, and excess salt from your diet. Now comes the fun part! The Blood Pressure Down plan is not only about what you should limit in your diet (salt and calories) but also about what you should add in.

Why is it that in populations that consume a primarily plant-based diet—high in fruits and vegetables—only 1 percent of people suffer from high blood pressure, compared to populations that consume diets high in processed foods and salt, where one in three has this disease?[1] Scientists think it has to do with the ratio of two minerals, each of which has a tremendous effect on your arteries: sodium and potassium. As you know, Western diets are extraordinarily high in blood-pressure-raising sodium—and it turns out they are equally low in potassium, the blood-pressure-lowering supermineral. This is a situation that I'll show you how to reverse through the addition of two delicious foods to your diet.

One of the fruits we'll add to your day is bananas. Bananas are the most popular fruit in the United States. They are a delicious, portable, and relatively inexpensive fruit filled with fiber as well as many vitamins and minerals. But on top of that, bananas are Mother Nature's sweet blood-pressure-lowering medicine, because of their potassium content—one banana packs a potassium punch of at least 450 mg.

Another fruit that we're going to add to your daily diet is the small but mighty kiwi fruit (also known as the Chinese gooseberry). This furry little egg-shaped fruit is named after the kiwi bird, the brown flightless bird that is New Zealand's national symbol. Open up the fruit and you are treated to a bright green, sweet-tasting flesh, with rows of tiny, crunchy black seeds. So what's so special about kiwi fruit? Kiwi is a nutrition powerhouse, with almost as much potassium as a banana for only half the calories.

Let's explore why potassium is your blood pressure's best friend.

THE POWER OF POTASSIUM

Americans have a mineral balance problem. As you learned in the last chapter, for decades we have been aware that eating too much salt is bad for blood pressure. But there is another equally important player in the blood pressure challenge—potassium. We don't eat nearly enough of this superb mineral, and our woefully inadequate intake of potassium-rich foods is taking its toll on our health. The reason for this mineral imbalance is—you guessed it—American's processed food obsession. Processing drastically changes the mineral makeup of natural foods, increasing sodium and decreasing potassium—a dietary manipulation that has dire health consequences.

Potassium: Sodium's Foe

Potassium is both a mineral and an electrolyte found naturally in the body. (Electrolytes are substances that can conduct electricity in your body.) Potassium and the other major mineral electrolytes, sodium, magnesium, and calcium, must be in precise equilibrium to maintain proper fluid balance and normal body functions such as nerve impulses, muscle contraction, and heart and brain activity.

When it comes to blood pressure regulation, sodium and potassium play separate but highly interactive biological roles in the body. Like Cain and Abel, sodium and potassium are brotherly enemies. As you know, a small amount of the mineral sodium is vital for health, but too much is harmful. Potassium is also an essential nutrient, and biologically it has the opposite effect on blood pressure.

There is a delicate balance of both minerals in the body. Most potassium resides within cells, whereas most sodium is located outside the cells, in the blood and lymph tissue. In the kidneys, dietary potassium and sodium have antagonistic physiological effects. In fact, increasing your dietary potassium intake can have a striking effect on urinary sodium excretion. When intake of sodium is high, the kidneys increase elimination of potassium. Conversely, eating more potassium will help decrease sodium levels by promoting cells to release sodium in exchange for potassium. The kidneys then excrete the sodium and excess water in your urine.

> Potassium exhibits strong blood-pressure-lowering effects on the blood vessels, which is why it enjoys a heart-healthy reputation.

In essence, potassium lowers blood pressure by balancing out the harmful effects of sodium. It works as a natural diuretic: the more potassium you eat, the more sodium and water you excrete in the urine. Scientists think that potassium also actively relaxes the blood vessels. But it's not just a high intake of dietary potassium that is the prescription for lowering your numbers; it's the relationship with its metabolic nemesis, sodium, that really matters.

To lower your blood pressure, you need to think beyond slashing salt. It's time to shift your attention to ingesting much, much more of Mother Nature's most powerful blood pressure medicine. Abundant scientific evidence has proven that a shortage

THREE KIWIS A DAY KEEPS BLOOD PRESSURE AT BAY

Kiwi, that funny-looking furry brown egg-shaped fruit, can actually make a dent in your blood pressure (and body weight) numbers. Three of these little fruits pack in 852 mg of potassium, 47 mg of magnesium, and 93 mg of calcium—and all these minerals for a measly 165 calories. When Norwegian researchers decided to conduct a kiwifruit experiment, they tested the effects of eating three kiwis a day in smokers with high blood pressure (using a randomized controlled clinical trial—the gold standard of experimental research) for a period of eight weeks. The results? Nothing short of miraculous: a drop in blood pressure of 10 mm Hg in the systolic number and 9 mm Hg in the diastolic number. Not only that, but the kiwi group showed a 15 percent reduction in blood clotting (platelet aggregation) and an 11 percent reduction in the activity of the main blood-pressure-raising enzyme, angiotensin-converting enzyme or ACE. (You may already take a prescription drug called an ACE inhibitor that lowers pressure in the same fashion.)

Source: Karlsen A, Svendsen M, Seljeflot I, et al. Kiwifruit decreases blood pressure and whole-blood platelet aggregation in male smokers. *J Hum Hypertens* 2012:1–5. DOI:10.1038/jhh.2011.116.

of potassium in the diet has a critical role in promoting high blood pressure. Indeed, restricting potassium intake has been proven to cause a substantial rise in blood pressure—even in people with normal blood pressure. A low potassium intake also ups your odds of suffering a stroke.

Loading up on potassium-rich foods is a key to regulating blood pressure and, outside of its relationship with sodium, can actually have a dramatic blood-pressure-lowering effect in and of itself. In fact, if you watch your sodium but fail to ingest the required amount of potassium, your blood pressure may not drop and you will be missing an important part of the picture. Unfortunately, most Americans are grossly deficient in their intake of this artery-friendly nutrient—according to the latest *Dietary Guidelines for Americans 2010* report, 97 percent of us do not achieve the recommended potassium intake.[2] In fact, potassium has made the report's list of the top six underconsumed nutrients of public concern (vitamins A, C, and K, fiber, and magnesium complete the list). Let's change that—read on to learn how to prop up your potassium intake to power down your blood pressure numbers.

The Balancing Act

When it comes to manipulating blood pressure with dietary minerals, it's all in the balance. Humans can regulate blood pressure simply by changing what they eat and altering the ratio of the powerful minerals sodium and potassium. Over the last half million years or so, salt was a rare commodity for humans, so our bodies developed mechanisms to conserve sodium and excrete potassium, which was always plentiful in the primitive diet. The adrenal hormone aldosterone conserves sodium and increases excretion of potassium, resulting in fluid retention and higher blood pressure. (Certain medications such as eplerenone work to block the action of this hormone, resulting in lowering of blood pressure.)

Fast-forward to the present day and the typical American way of eating, with our reliance on packaged convenience foods, fast foods, chips, and ordering off a menu. The result is an unnatural overload of sodium and a deficit of potassium. The chronic imbalance of sodium and potassium ingestion wreaks havoc on your system, with elevated blood pressure as the symptom.

How Much Potassium Is Enough?

The solution is to revert back to the ratio of minerals that the body was designed to consume. The simultaneous reduction in sodium and increase in potassium will heal the arteries and reverse the damage. You know that you should be getting no more than 1,500 mg of sodium per day. Combined with this, just how much potassium does one need to consume to achieve blood pressure reduction benefits?

You need to take in at least three times the amount of potassium as sodium—that's the finding from the famed DASH diet studies. In the original study, subjects consumed approximately 4,400 mg/day of potassium, which lowered blood pressure by an average of 2.8/1.1 mm Hg in people with normal blood pressure and by an average of 7.2/2.8 mm Hg in people with high blood pressure.[3,4]

The current American Heart Association recommendation for potassium intake is now 4,700 mg/day, a value based on recent clin-

THE UNCHECKED EPIDEMIC AMONG AFRICAN AMERICANS

High blood pressure is killing off the African American community at an unprecedented rate. Approximately 40 percent of African Americans have high blood pressure—the highest rate of any group in the United States. African Americans progress from prehypertension to full-blown high blood pressure faster than white Americans and have considerably more complications from high blood pressure, such as heart attacks, stroke, and kidney disease. Blacks are hospitalized for high blood pressure about five times as often as whites, with the highest rates of admittance among low-income women living on the fringes of large metropolitan areas or in the Northeast.

Why is this so? It has been hypothesized that blacks may be more salt sensitive and consume less potassium than white Americans. In fact, potassium has a greater blood-pressure-lowering effect in blacks compared to whites, and the DASH diet was scientifically proven to be particularly beneficial among this segment of the population.

Sources: Agency for Health Care Research and Quality. Blacks hospitalized for high blood pressure five times more often than whites. *Agency News and Notes* 2010. Sept; Douglas JG, Bakris GL, Epstein M, et al. Management of high blood pressure in African Americans—consensus statement of the Hypertension in African Americans Working Group of the International Society on Hypertension in Blacks. *Arch Int Med* 2003;163(5):525–541; Whelton PK, He J, Cutler JA, et al. Effects of oral potassium on blood pressure: meta-analysis of randomized controlled clinical trials. *JAMA* 1997;277(20):1624–1632.

ical trials.[5] This is the amount American adults need to keep blood pressure in check, blunt the harmful effects of sodium, and reduce the risk of bone loss and kidney stones. The reality is that most of us fall far short, with the average American eating just about half the recommended amount.[6] Take control of your health and begin today to reap the superb health benefits of eating more natural, fresh, unprocessed foods with a balanced intake of potassium and sodium.

THE BENEFITS OF DIETARY POTASSIUM

Be Savvy About Supplements

Most experts agree that it is best to get your potassium in the form of food. But what about supplements? Elemental potassium alone tastes bitter, so supplement companies add chloride to make it more palatable. And although the evidence is robust that a high dietary

---

DIETARY POTASSIUM CUTS NEED FOR BLOOD PRESSURE DRUGS IN HALF

Got high blood pressure and taking meds to control it? Increasing your intake of dietary potassium from natural foods can cut your medication needs in half. That's the finding from a one-year randomized clinical trial published in the prestigious *Annals of Internal Medicine*. Forty-seven patients on prescription medication for previously diagnosed high blood pressure were randomly assigned to one of two groups: high dietary potassium intake or a customary diet. (The high-potassium diet was achieved by increasing the consumption of vegetables and legumes and by moderately increasing fresh fruit intake.) By the end of the study, the large majority of the patients on the potassium diet were able to control their pressure using less than 50 percent of the drug dose they were initially taking.

Source: Siani A, Strazzullo P, Giacco A, et al. Increasing the dietary potassium intake reduces the need for antihypertensive medication. *Ann Int Med* 1991;115(10):753–759.

intake of potassium lowers blood pressure, data from individual trials examining the influence of potassium chloride on blood pressure in hypertensive subjects have been inconsistent.[7]

The takeaway? Potassium that does *not* contain chloride, such as potassium found naturally in the foods recommended in this chapter, offers larger benefits for reducing blood pressure than potassium in supplement form.[8] Need more reasons why you should choose to eat potassium-rich foods over popping supplements? At the cell wall, the natural form of potassium promotes a greater exchange of sodium ions than does potassium chloride. To get your blood pressure down, our goal is to alter the exchange of ions at the cell wall, to increase the amount of potassium entering the cells and sodium exiting. More potassium in and sodium out of the cells results in a greater blood-pressure-lowering effect.

POTASSIUM: POWER DOWN PRESSURE, BUILD UP BONES

A high-potassium diet is not just good for your blood pressure—it's also good for your bones. Unprocessed fruits and vegetables contain what are called bicarbonate precursors, substances that favorably affect acid-base metabolism in the body. A less acidic milieu reduces the risk of kidney stones and bone loss. Meat, milk, and cereal products also contain potassium, they but do not have the same positive effect on acid-base metabolism.

Source: Institute of Medicine of the National Academies. Dietary reference intakes: water, potassium, sodium, chloride and sulfate 2004. Feb 11.

Diet Makes a Big Difference When It Comes to Potassium

The fact is that diets brimming with fresh, unprocessed fruits and vegetables are potassium rich and sodium poor—just what we're after! For example, an orange contains zero sodium and 326 mg potassium (with 62 calories). Conversely, the typical American diet, based on processed foods, provides a sodium overload and is sparse in potassium. For example, an Arby's breakfast Ham 'n Cheese Croissant contains 870 mg of sodium and zero potassium (and 350 calories). It's no wonder that we have an epidemic of high blood pressure and obesity in this country! The simple act of eating two kiwi fruits and a large banana every day will help you make a nice dent in your daily potassium goal.

Change the Ratio, Pay the Consequences

What would happen if you took an entire genetically homogeneous population, free of high blood pressure and subsisting on a diet of natural, unprocessed foods, and moved half the people to an urbanized Western society with all the trappings of modern life? This is exactly what happened when more than half the Tokelau society migrated from the tropical atolls where they had lived for centuries to the New Zealand mainland after a disastrous hurricane in 1966. The nonmigrant population remained in three villages, living a traditional Polynesian lifestyle and eating a natural-foods diet. A group of scientists compared the migrants to the nonmigrants only five years after the migration.

What happened? As you can probably predict by now, the migrants' blood pressure (and body weight) shot up dramatically as their dietary potassium-to-sodium ratio plummeted.[9]

When It Comes to Blood Pressure, You Are What You Eat

As you have learned, a high-potassium, low-sodium dietary intake pattern is best for getting your blood pressure down. Conversely, not eating enough dietary potassium increases both systolic and diastolic blood pressure numbers in people with high blood pressure and even in those with normal blood pressure readings.[10]

Your pressure truly reflects what you eat. Go to the supermarket and load up on potassium power foods listed in the table on pages 114–115. Pile your plate with them and you will soon reap the phenomenal rewards of natural potassium!

Potassium Power Foods

Food	Serving Size	Potassium (mg)
Baked potato	1 medium	1,080
Pistachios	¾ C	1,000
Avocado	1 medium	975
Swiss chard, raw	1 C	961
Prunes, dried	4 large	940
Spinach, cooked	1 C	839
Apricots, dried	½ C	750
Sweet Potato, baked	1 medium	694
Banana	1 medium	569
Figs, dried	½ C	500
White beans, cooked	½ C	500
Molasses	1 Tb	498
Brussels sprouts, boiled	1 C	495
Halibut, cooked	3 oz	490
Lima beans, cooked	½ C	477
Broccoli, steamed	1 C	457
Snapper, cooked	3 oz	444
Cantaloupe, chopped	1 C	427
Grouper, cooked	3 oz	404
Asparagus, cooked	1 C	404
Tomato, sliced	1 medium	400
Pinto beans, cooked	½ C	400
Trout, cooked	3 oz	394
Honeydew, chopped	1 C	388
Cucumber, peeled	1 large	381
Salmon, wild, cooked	3 oz	369
Carrots, chopped, cooked	1 C	366
Raisins	⅓ C	363
Mango, raw	1 medium	348
Romaine lettuce, chopped	2 C	325
Dates	5 medium	324
Red peppers, chopped, raw	1 C	314

Food	Serving Size	Potassium (mg)
Celery, raw	1 C	312
Cauliflower, raw	1 C	303
Kale, cooked, chopped	1 C	296
Turnip greens, cooked, chopped	1 C	292
Peach	1 medium	285
Kiwi fruit	1 large	284
Nectarine	1 medium	273
Lentils, cooked	½ C	269
Green peppers, chopped, raw	1 C	261
Strawberries	1 C	254
Orange	1 medium	237
Blackberries	1 C	233
Lean beef, cooked	3 oz	224
Mushrooms, white, raw	1 C	223
Peanut butter	2 Tb	214
Pear	1 medium	198
Green beans, cooked	½ C	187
Watermelon, chopped	1 C	176
Zucchini, cooked, chopped	½ C	173
Paprika	1 Tb	164
Cocoa powder, unsweetened	2 Tb	152
Chervil, dried	1 Tb	95
Grapes	10 grapes	93
Blueberries	½ C	63
Egg	1 egg	55
Basil. dried	1 Tb	50
Coriander, dried	1 Tb	50
Tarragon, dried	1 Tb	50
Cheddar cheese	1 oz	28

PROTECTIVE POWER OF POTASSIUM: STRONG SCIENCE

Increasing Potassium and Reducing Salt Prevents Strokes

Eating at least twice as much potassium as sodium can not only cut your pressure down to size, it can also shave the odds of suffering a debilitating stroke. That was the result of an Italian study, published in the *Journal of the American College of Cardiology*, the largest meta-analysis so far to examine the impact of potassium intake on vascular health.[11] Researchers pulled data about potassium and cardiovascular disease from eleven large-scale association trials, which included a total of nearly 250,000 men and women. The findings? People who ate about 1,600 mg more potassium per day had a 21 percent lower risk of stroke and also tended to have a lower risk of any form of cardiovascular disease. The scientists concluded that adding potassium-rich foods to our daily diet in conjunction with cutting salt intake could prevent as many as 1,155,000 worldwide stroke deaths per year.

In with Potassium, Out with Sodium: More Science Behind the Suggestion

Still not convinced about the power of potassium? Let's take a look at research published in the *Archives of Internal Medicine*, taken from the long-term Trials of Hypertension Prevention (TOHP) study, which once again shows how important it is to focus on the balance of sodium and potassium, rather than on either of these two minerals alone.[12] Scientists examined the urine of 2,275 middle-aged overweight men and women with prehypertension. (Sodium/potassium urinary excretion is a scientific method used to estimate the amounts of sodium and potassium typically consumed in the diet, and is a far more valid assessment of actual levels of sodium and potassium intake than relying on patients to report their own intake.) Results showed that over a period of ten to fifteen years, a low potassium-to-sodium ratio was the strongest link to increased risk of heart attack and stroke. And no surprise here: the scientists concluded that the ideal dietary strategy for lowering blood pressure and cutting risk of heart attacks and stroke is to eat potassium-rich foods such as fruits and vegetables, as well as cutting back on salt.

LOW-POTASSIUM, HIGH-SODIUM DIET
DOUBLES RISK OF EARLY DEATH

Another recent study in the *Archives of Internal Medicine* clarified the joint effect of sodium and potassium intake on mortality. The investigation was based on the Third National Health and Nutrition Examination Survey (1988–2006), a long-term study of a nationally representative sample of more than twelve thousand American adults followed for a period of fifteen years. Data from the survey illustrated a significant relationship between both potassium and sodium intake and health. People who consumed a low-potassium, high-sodium diet had a 50 percent increased risk of dying during the study period (from any cause), and nearly twice the risk of death from heart disease compared to those eating a high-potassium, low-sodium diet. Conversely, study participants who consumed 4,069 milligrams of potassium a day (close to the 4,700 in our Blood Pressure Down plan) had half the risk of death from all causes compared to those who took in 1,793 milligrams a day (a little less than the average intake).

The major implication of these findings is that a diet balanced in both micronutrients is important. The higher the potassium intake and the lower the sodium intake, the longer you live free of disease. The authors suggested that an increase in potassium intake accompanied by a reduction in sodium intake could achieve greater health benefits than restricting sodium alone.

Source: Yang Q, Liu T, Kuklina EV, et al. Sodium and potassium intake and mortality among US adults: prospective data from the Third National Health and Nutrition Examination Survey. *Arch Intern Med* 2011;171(13):1183–1191.

The huge INTERSALT study of more than ten thousand men and women, ages twenty to fifty-nine, from fifty-two centers around the world, also examined the relationship between blood pressure and twenty-four-hour urinary excretion of sodium and potassium.[13] The study found that those people who had the highest ratio of potassium to sodium in their diet were at lowest risk of dying from a heart attack or stroke. Conversely, those with diets containing a low potassium intake and a high sodium intake had a 46 percent higher risk of dying. The authors suggest that a high ratio of potassium to sodium in the diet could blunt the rise in blood pressure that often accompanies aging.

HOW DOES POTASSIUM LOWER BLOOD PRESSURE?

The interaction between sodium and potassium in the body is the dominant environmental cause of high blood pressure.[14] Here is how changing your intake of these minerals affects your blood pressure numbers.

Method of attack #1: Piling on the potassium affects your arteries where it counts, deep down in the inner lining of the arterial wall. The endothelial cells serve as the control center for producing nitric oxide, the calming chemical that relaxes the vessels. More potassium in your body means those cells produce more nitric oxide, which relaxes blood vessels and thereby lowers blood pressure. More potassium also activates potassium channels, or gateways into the cell. This helps the blood vessels dilate, further decreasing pressure.[15]

Method of attack #2: As you know, not enough potassium and too much sodium increases blood pressure and causes fluid retention. Changing the ratio by bumping up your potassium levels is like taking a water pill: it promotes the release of extra fluids and sodium through the urine, thereby lowering the pressure on your artery walls.

Method of attack #3: A potassium shortage triggers your body's sympathetic nervous system, which increases blood pressure. The activity of the renin-angiotensin system is also stimulated, meaning more renin (the vessel-squeezing enzyme manufactured by the kidneys) is produced and pressure rises even more. (Recall from Chapter Two that an overactive renin-angiotensin system leads to tightened blood vessels and retention of sodium and water.) Increasing the intake of potassium acts like taking two drugs: Valium and an ACE inhibitor. The result is a suppression of the sympathetic nervous system, suppression of renin output, calming of the nerves, and dilation of your blood vessels—all of which serve to lower your pressure.

Method of attack #4: The combination of not enough potassium with excess salt intake alters the mineral exchange and reabsorption that happens in the kidneys—the primary organ affecting blood pressure numbers. This makes your body retain more sodium and excrete more potassium, raising your blood pressure. Increase the potassium and lower the salt, and the kidney's filtering actions will go back to normal (sodium excretion and potassium retention).

POTASSIUM CAUTION

There are a few important caveats regarding potassium consumption. Some people, such as those with diabetes or chronic kidney disease and those taking medications that affect potassium balance (including potassium-sparing diuretics such as spironolactone), should not ingest too much potassium. If you have a medical condition that impairs kidney function or if you are on a medication that hinders potassium excretion, then you must restrict your intake of potassium to avoid adverse cardiac effects from hyperkalemia (an abnormally high concentration of potassium in the bloodstream).[16] Also, many foods high in potassium are rich in vitamin K as well. If you take blood-thinning medications such as warfarin, your doctor may ask you to limit your intake of vitamin K, which can interfere with the action of anticoagulant drugs. If you fall into any of these categories, be sure to check with your personal physician before bumping up your daily dose of potassium.

FILLING THE PRESCRIPTION

Head for the greengrocer's and harness the power of potassium for blood pressure control. Fill your fridge with the potassium power foods listed on pages 114–115. Carry around the Minerals Pocket Charts (Appendix 6), and when you see any of the foods listed there, eat them! In so doing, you will be taking a powerful step in pushing those millimeters down.

TEN TIPS FOR ADDING POTASSIUM INTO YOUR DAY

1. Eat the following foods daily: 1 banana, 2 kiwis, a 10-ounce package of fresh spinach (which cooks down to a very small quantity), 2 cups nonfat yogurt, a can of low-sodium V8, and a cup of homemade soy milk cocoa (recipe on page 265). If you squeeze them all in, you are good to go on all mineral counts!

2. Order unseasoned grilled salmon and baked potatoes (salt-free) at restaurants (bring your own salt substitute for the potato and use lemon juice for the fish).

3. Snack on salt-free pistachios.

4. Use avocado as a sandwich spread in lieu of mayonnaise.

5. Fry your omelet (made with egg whites, of course!) with added spinach.

6. Eat cantaloupe cubes (available precut at the grocery store).

7. Eat potassium power salads: dark leafy greens, red peppers, broccoli, cauliflower, tomato, carrots, avocado, rinsed white beans, and low-sodium tuna.

---

8. Eat banana and peanut butter sandwiches (I like the Better'n Peanut Butter low-sodium, reduced-calorie brand) on 100 percent whole-wheat low-sodium bread.

9. Add dried figs, prunes, and apricots to your morning bowl of oatmeal.

10. Fill your fruit bowl with oranges, bananas, and kiwi and snack on them throughout the day.

Potassium is truly your blood vessels' best friend. Get enough of it in your day from healthful fresh, unprocessed whole foods and you can make a significant dent in your blood pressure numbers and protect your heart. Understand that the interplay of sodium and potassium in the diet is the critical factor. To prevent, treat, and reverse high blood pressure, you must make a concerted effort to shake the sodium *and* power up the potassium—a goal that requires perseverance in a world where the food supply is increasingly processed.

Potassium is just one of the trio of mineral superheroes that interact in your body to curb your millimeters of mercury. Let's discover the second player in your arsenal of disease-fighting nutrients, the magnificent mineral magnesium.

7

Step 4: Eat Spinach

℞ Eat 500 mg of Magnesium Every Day

Popeye was right when he told you to eat your spinach! Spinach packs a nutritional double whammy: it's loaded not just with potassium but also with magnesium, the second blood-pressure-lowering mineral superstar. Magnesium is potassium's mineral "twin"—the two elements are so tightly bound metabolically that it is difficult to maintain an adequate level of potassium in the cells if you are not eating enough magnesium, no matter how much potassium you manage to eat. Because magnesium is such a key player in reducing those millimeters of mercury, eating foods rich in magnesium is therefore an essential component of the Blood Pressure Down plan. So read on to learn just what and how much you need to consume to take the correct "dosage" of one of Mother Nature's most powerful blood-pressure-lowering mineral medicines.

THE ORIGINAL BLOOD-PRESSURE-LOWERING
MINERAL MACHINE

As you know, the famed DASH diet studies provided the first convincing scientific evidence that a nonpharmaceutical lifestyle treatment could significantly reduce blood pressure. In those studies, a special trio of minerals—potassium, magnesium, and calcium, taken in food rather than as supplements—were proven to be especially valuable for blood pressure management. See the table below for a summary of the DASH diet (more information about DASH can be found on the website of the National Heart, Lung, and Blood Institute, www.nhlbi.nih.gov).

Nuts and Bolts of the DASH
(Dietary Approaches to Stop Hypertension) Diet

Food Group	Number of Servings			Sample Servings of Food
	1,200-calorie diet	2,000-calorie diet	2,600-calorie diet	
Grains and grain products	6 per day	6–8 per day	10–11 per day	1 slice bread ½ C dry cereal ½ C cooked pasta
Vegetables	3–4 per day	4–5 per day	5–6 per day	1 C raw green leafy vegetables ½ C cooked vegetables ½ C vegetable juice
Fruit	4 per day	4–5 per day	5–6 per day	1 medium fruit ¼ C dried fruit ½ C fruit juice
Fat-free or low-fat dairy	2–3 per day	2–3 per day	3 per day	1 C fat-free milk 1½ oz reduced-fat cheese
Meat, poultry, fish	3–6 per day	6 or less per day	6 per day	1 oz broiled or baked lean meats, skinless poultry, or fish 1 egg
Nuts, seeds, beans	3 per week	4–5 per week	1 per day	1½ oz nuts ½ C cooked beans 2 Tb peanut butter
Added fats and oils	2 per day	2–3 per day	3 per day	1 t oil 1 Tb regular salad dressing 2 Tb light salad dressing
Sweets and added sugars	0	5 or less per week	2 or less per day	1 Tb sugar 1 Tb jelly or jam ½ C sorbet

It should be noted that it is consumption of the *whole* DASH dietary pattern that is most effective for reducing blood pressure, not just any of the individual minerals on its own.

MANAGING YOUR PRESSURE WITH MAGNESIUM

What Is Magnesium?

Magnesium is the fourth most abundant mineral in the body (following calcium, phosphorus, and potassium). It is an essential nutrient for life, present in all cells. The correct balance of magnesium is vital for well-being and general good health. Magnesium is a biologically active mineral electrolyte. About half of our total magnesium stores are locked up in our bones and teeth. The rest is located in muscles and soft tissues, with just 1 percent floating in our bloodstream. Magnesium is essential for proper metabolism—it is needed in more than three hundred biochemical reactions. It gets excreted in your urine via your kidneys, or retained in the body to make up for a low dietary intake.

Magnesium helps control your blood pressure in several ways.[1] First, it has a direct effect on the proper functioning of the endothelium, the inner arterial wall. (Recall that a dysfunctional endothelium is the root cause of high blood pressure.) Magnesium has direct antioxidant and anti-inflammatory properties that attenuate damage to the delicate endothelial cells. Second, magnesium helps regulate the transport of other minerals—calcium, potassium, and sodium—across cell walls. It combines with the other minerals in the body to achieve the delicate balance that is vital to regulating your blood pressure.

As you know, your body—and, in fact, all higher life-forms—require a subtle and complex electrolyte balance for normal functioning. Our bodies have numerous mechanisms that keep the mineral concentrations under tight control, and magnesium is a crucial piece of the puzzle—it works alongside calcium and potassium to balance the sodium in your body. A shortage of magnesium in your diet throws off the balance of sodium, potassium, and calcium, which causes the blood vessels to constrict.[2] Following the Blood Pressure Down plan will help you keep the mineral balance to get your pressure where you want it to be (Figure 7.1).

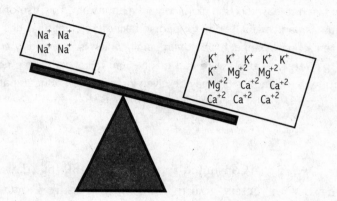

Figure 7.1 A robust dietary intake of three specific minerals: potassium (4,700 mg/day), magnesium (500 mg/ day) and calcium (1,200 mg/day) is required to offset your sodium intake (1,500 mg/day) and for getting and keeping your blood pressure down.

You already know that a diet with too much sodium and not enough potassium wreaks havoc. But too little magnesium also throws off your mineral metabolism. Magnesium depletion drains potassium—the number one blood-pressure-regulating mineral— from the body. So no matter how much potassium you eat, it's virtually impossible to keep enough in your bloodstream unless you have enough magnesium, too.

How Much Magnesium Is Enough?

The recommended daily intake of magnesium is 320 mg/day for women and 420 mg/day for men. Americans are woefully short in their intake of dietary magnesium, with 48 percent of us failing to consume anywhere near this amount.[3] And we know from the DASH studies that even the RDA is not enough to contribute to lower blood pressure numbers. The most successful group in the

MEDICINAL MAGIC OF MAGNESIUM

Magnesium is great for your blood pressure, and it also has bonus health benefits. You may have heard that many over-the-counter laxatives, used to ease constipation, contain magnesium. This use of magnesium is particularly helpful for people taking prescription drugs such as the calcium channel blocker verapamil, which is notoriously constipating. Were you also aware that magnesium helps maintain a normal heart rhythm? Magnesium may be given intravenously to heart patients to reduce the risk of atrial fibrillation or irregular heartbeat.

original DASH trial consumed approximately 480 mg/day of magnesium, so your dietary goal in the Blood Pressure Down plan is 500 mg magnesium per day. Dig into the magnesium power foods found in the table on pages 127–128 and you can easily get your 500 mg daily dose of magnesium and then some.

WAKE UP AND SMELL THE COFFEE!

This might be the best nutrition news since dark chocolate! Coffee is the number one source of antioxidants in the American diet, linked with reduced risk of developing a number of diseases such as diabetes, heart disease, Parkinson's, and Alzheimer's. Coffee is loaded with magnesium as well as a family of potent plant chemicals called chlorogenic acids (CGAs), the main components of a type of antioxidant called polyphenols. Scientists have shown that the consumption of CGAs can reduce blood pressure by increasing production of the all-important blood-pressure-regulating chemical nitric oxide, which helps relax artery walls. One caveat before you down your cup of joe: be sure to watch the caffeine intake, as excessive amounts can actually raise your pressure temporarily.

Source: Zhao Y, Wang J, Ballevre O, et al. Antihypertensive effects and mechanisms of chlorogenic acids. *Hypertens Res* 2011;35:370–374.

Magnesium Power Foods

Food	Serving Size	Magnesium (mg)
Cocoa powder	1 C	428
Brazil nuts	½ C	250
Pine nuts	½ C	170
Pumpkin seeds	1 oz	156
Spinach, boiled	1 C	157
Swiss chard	1 C	151
White beans, cooked	1 C	134
Black beans, cooked	1 C	120
Oatmeal, cooked	1 C	112
Corn	½ C	106
Artichokes	1 C	101
Edamame	1 C	99
Halibut, cooked	3 oz	91
Lima beans, cooked	1 C	81
Chickpeas, cooked	1 C	79
Almonds, raw	24	76
Dates, raw, chopped	1 C	63
Quinoa, cooked	½ C	59
Wild salmon, cooked	½ fillet	59
Okra, cooked	1 C	58
Tahini	1 Tb	58
Scallops, cooked	6 large	55
Tuna, broiled	3 oz	54
Wild rice, cooked	1 C	52
Pollock	1 fillet	49
Peanut butter	2 Tb	49
Molasses	1 Tb	48
Soy milk	1 C	47
Peas, cooked	1 C	46
Walnuts	14 halves	44

Food	Serving Size	Magnesium (mg)
Brown rice, cooked	½ C	42
Flaxseeds	1 Tb	39
Tofu	¼ block	37
Sesame seeds	1 oz	37
Cod, cooked	3 oz	36
Avocado	½ C puree	35
Lentils, cooked	½ C	36
Banana	1 medium	34
Mustard seed, yellow	1 Tb	33
Celery seed	1 Tb	29
Chicken breast, cooked	3.5 oz	27
Kale, boiled	1 C	24
Kiwi	1 medium	23
Broccoli, raw	1 C	22
Cumin seed, whole	1 Tb	22
Curry powder	1 Tb	16
Dried coriander	1 Tb	14
Turmeric, ground	1 Tb	13
Paprika	1 Tb	13
Pepper, black	1 Tb	12
Sage, ground	1 Tb	9
Parsley, dried	1 Tb	4
Basil, fresh, chopped	2 Tb	3
Basil, dried	1 tsp	2

SCIENTIFIC MUSCLE BEHIND MAGNESIUM

We know from numerous large observational studies that people who eat a diet rich in magnesium develop high blood pressure at a much lower rate.[4] A recent review of forty-four clinical trials concluded that 486 mg of magnesium a day is necessary to significantly lower blood pressure.[5] The Joint National Committee on Preven-

MAGNESIUM CUTS RISK OF DEATH
FROM A HEART ATTACK IN HALF

Hot off the presses is a new large-scale observational study out of Japan linking dietary magnesium intake with better heart health and longevity. Nearly fifty-nine thousand healthy Japanese people were followed for fifteen years. The scientists found that those people with the highest dietary intake of magnesium had a 50 percent reduction in their risk of death from cardiovascular disease (heart attack and stroke). According to the researchers, magnesium's heart-healthy benefit is linked to its ability to improve blood pressure, suppress irregular heartbeats, and inhibit inflammation.

Source: Zhang W, Iso H, Ohira T, et al. Associations of dietary magnesium intake with mortality from cardiovascular disease: the JACC study. *Atherosclerosis* 2012;221(2):587–595.

tion, Detection, Evaluation, and Treatment of High Blood Pressure agrees, officially recommending diets high in magnesium for individuals with hypertension.[6] One question that many scientists ponder is whether magnesium alone improves blood pressure or whether magnesium-rich diets lower pressure simply because they are also rich in other healthful nutrients such as potassium, fiber, and plant antioxidants. The verdict is still out, but this question should hammer home the fact that a single nutrient is *not* the secret to health. Your best medicine is obtaining your nutrients from a varied, healthful diet.

Can't I Just Take Magnesium Supplements?

Popping magnesium pills doesn't appear to do the trick. A powerful meta-analysis of twenty randomized clinical trials found that taking magnesium supplements (at a median dosage of 370 mg/day) had no effect on blood pressure.[7] Boosting dietary intake of magnesium the old-fashioned way—from food—appears to be the most effective blood-pressure-lowering method.

MAGNESIUM SLASHES RISK OF STROKE

A recent well-designed meta-analysis reveals that eating magnesium may just be the best medicine for reducing your risk of stroke. Pooling data from seven large-scale studies of more than 240,000 participants, Swedish researchers concluded that every 100 mg per day increase in dietary magnesium was associated with a 9 percent reduction in risk of stroke.

Source: Larsson SC, Orsini N, Wolk A. Dietary magnesium intake and risk of stroke: a meta-analysis of prospective studies. *Am J Clin Nutr* 2012;95(2):362–366.

HOW DOES MAGNESIUM LOWER BLOOD PRESSURE?

Aside from its strong association with potassium, magnesium also soothes the arteries and lowers blood pressure through several other processes. Dietary magnesium is a biologically active mineral that is good for the heart, the brain, and the blood vessels. Read on to learn how this magnificent mineral works its medicinal magic.

Method of attack #1: Magnesium regulates calcium's movement across the membranes of the smooth muscle cells deep within the artery walls. If your body doesn't have enough magnesium, too much calcium enters the smooth muscle cells, which causes the cells to contract, putting a squeeze on the arteries and raising blood pressure.[8] In this way, magnesium is actually Mother Nature's natural calcium channel blocker. It acts in a fashion very similar to that of synthetic pharmacological calcium antagonists such as diltiazem, which blocks calcium and relaxes and widens the blood vessels.[9]

Method of attack #2: Magnesium soothes the muscles in your blood vessels, acting like yoga for the arteries. It has been scientifically proven that magnesium ions actively promote cellular relaxation by offsetting the electrical ion exchange activity.[10]

Method of attack #3: Magnesium therapy decreases the

potential for dangerous arrhythmias, or irregular heartbeats, which can be fatal in heart patients. Magnesium helps the heart cells maintain their intracellular potassium level, which strengthens the ability of the heart muscle to transmit electrical currents and contract properly.[11]

Method of attack #4: Magnesium helps regulate the renin-angiotensin-aldosterone system. Recall that aldosterone is the "salt keeper" hormone that causes your kidneys to retain sodium and water, raising your blood pressure. Less aldosterone means lower blood pressure. Magnesium curbs secretion of aldosterone by the adrenal glands, and blood pressure drops.[12]

Method of attack #5: Magnesium is anti-inflammatory—you can think of it functioning almost like cortisone cream on the inner arterial wall. As you know, one of the reasons high blood pressure develops is because the inner layer of the arteries, the endothelium, becomes inflamed and dysfunctional. A high intake of magnesium from food is associated with lower amounts of the inflammatory markers in the blood that indicate systemic inflammation and endothelial dysfunction.[13]

MAGNESIUM CAUTION

If you are taking diuretics, have diabetes, or drink excessive amounts of alcohol, you may be especially prone to developing a magnesium (and potassium) deficiency—all the more reason to follow the healthy eating advice set forth in these pages. But it is important to note a few key caveats regarding magnesium consumption.

There is no designated maximum for the amount of magnesium that you can eat—there is no evidence that magnesium from food sources, in any amount, can be toxic. But there *is* a toxicity problem associated with magnesium *supplements*. High doses of magnesium in supplement form can have side effects including loss of appetite, muscle weakness, diarrhea, and nausea. The bottom line: do not take magnesium supplements unless your doctor prescribes them.

You should also be mindful of magnesium antagonists—certain foods, drugs, and other minerals that can interfere with the absorption of magnesium. For example, high doses of supplemental zinc and high protein intake interfere with magnesium absorption, as does excessive laxative use and use of certain oral contraceptives. Be sure to ask your doctor about magnesium and drug interactions.

FILLING THE PRESCRIPTION

To consume the Blood Pressure Down goal of at least 500 mg daily, you will need to munch that magnesium! Head for your supermarket and harness the power of this miracle mineral. Fill your fridge and pantry with the magnesium power foods listed on pages 127–128. Carry around the Minerals Pocket Charts (Appendix 6), and when you see any of the foods listed there, eat them! In so doing, you will be taking another powerful, additive step in pushing those millimeters down.

TEN TIPS FOR ADDING MAGNESIUM INTO YOUR DAY

1. Wake up to your morning cup of joe. Coffee and espresso are excellent sources of magnesium. (If you tend to drink a lot of coffee, consider switching to decaf.)
2. Make a nightly cup of hot cocoa using unsweetened dark cocoa powder and light soy milk.
3. Sauté up some spinach with pine nuts and raisins (cook with extra-virgin olive oil).
4. Bake with molasses. Blackstrap molasses packs a good amount of magnesium. You can also use it to add nutrition to your oatmeal or even coffee.

---

5. Eat nuts! Unless you are allergic, these are a wonderful high-magnesium food.
6. Snack on roasted pumpkin seeds (usually available in the supermarket in the snack food section, next to the nuts). Just 1 ounce contains a whopping 75 mg of magnesium.
7. Use tofu in cooking. Half a cup packs 50 mg of magnesium for just 88 calories.
8. Get some Latin flavor in your cooking and serve black beans as a side dish. They contain a massive amount of magnesium (120 mg per cup).
9. Cook up some buckwheat pancakes on Sunday mornings. Buckwheat flour boasts 301 mg of magnesium per cup.
10. Order halibut next time you eat at a seafood restaurant. Halibut not only packs in 170 mg of magnesium per half a filet, it also contains a nice amount of heart-healthy omega-3 fat.

Magnesium has sometimes been called the "orphan nutrient," a forgotten mineral that has been studied considerably less than calcium and flies below the general public's radar.[14] But this is changing as more and more scientists are jumping on the magnesium bandwagon. We know that a magnesium-deficient diet is a major factor contributing to the development of many diseases—most notably high blood pressure.

Magnesium is just the second of the trio of mineral superheroes that interact in your body to curb your millimeters of mercury. Let's discover the third and last major mineral player in your arsenal of disease-fighting electrolytes, the phenomenal blood-pressure-busting mineral calcium.

Step 5: Eat Yogurt

℞ Eat 1,200 mg of Calcium Every Day

Yogurt has a long and colorful history. Until the early 1900s, it was a staple food in the Russian empire. At the time, scientists attributed the unusually long life span of Bulgarian peasants—many of whom lived well past the century mark—to the regular consumption of yogurt. Whether or not you believe the longevity lore surrounding yogurt, the fact is that this underappreciated health food is one of your most powerful blood-pressure-lowering tools. Yogurt is simply packed with nutrients: "predigested proteins" for easy absorption; live friendly bacteria for boosting immunity and colon health; as much potassium as in a banana; and more calcium than a glass of milk. This brings us to the crux of this chapter: the importance of calcium, the last of the three mineral superstars that you need to ingest in large quantities to get your blood pressure down.

The importance of eating enough calcium for strengthening our bones and teeth has been drilled into our heads for decades. Calcium has grabbed headlines as a mineral idol, shining under a halo of publicity. But not so fast! What about the recent stains on calcium's reputation of late, with scientists suggesting that calcium supplements actually *increase* your risk of heart attack? How much is too much? And does calcium help or hinder your blood pressure management regimen? Let's sort nutrition fact from fiction. Read on as we weigh the pros and cons of consuming calcium for getting your blood pressure down.

One thing is for sure: populations that don't eat much calcium have high rates of high blood pressure.[1] Conversely, eating lots of calcium-rich foods can have a dramatic blood-pressure-lowering impact on your numbers. How do we know this? Once again, we hark back to the famed DASH diet studies to find out how dietary calcium curbs those millimeters of mercury. The first DASH study clearly showed that consuming calcium-rich, low-fat or fat-free dairy foods—as part of a diet high in fruits and vegetables—doubled the blood-pressure-lowering results observed with the fruit-and-vegetable diet alone.[2] The bottom line: for maximum blood-pressure-lowering results, get your fruits and veggies *and* your calcium.

THE BLOOD PRESSURE BENEFITS OF CALCIUM

What Is Calcium?

Calcium is the most abundant mineral in the human body, with 99 percent stored away in our bones and teeth. Our bones act as a calcium reservoir, supplying calcium to the bloodstream when supplies diminish and storing excess when the blood value is too high. The 1 percent of calcium floating in the bloodstream and not trapped in the skeleton is vital for regulating critical metabolic processes. And calcium is intricately involved in blood vessel contraction and dilation, which controls your blood pressure. Ingesting the right amount of calcium (not too much and not too little) on a daily basis is essential for optimal blood pressure regulation. Why? If we don't get enough in our diet, the only other way the body can get the calcium it needs is by pulling it out of our bones.

How Much Is Enough?

According to the latest government recommendations, most American adults should be eating 1,000 to 1,200 mg of calcium per day. How are we doing? Many of us—especially adolescent girls, postmenopausal women, and elderly men and women, the groups who need it most—are coming up woefully short. The principal nutritional deficit that characterizes Americans with high blood pressure is calcium.[3] African Americans particularly tend to come up short on this blood-pressure-friendly mineral, which may be one reason why high blood pressure is epidemic among this segment of the population.[4]

For lowering blood pressure, the daily goal for calcium appears to be in the 1,200 mg range. The DASH study's most successful experimental group increased their dietary calcium intake to approximately 1,265 mg/day, consuming a daily average of two low-fat dairy products.[5] The "combination diet," rich in fruit, vegetables, *and* dairy products, lowered systolic blood pressure by 5.5 mm Hg and diastolic blood pressure by 3.0 mm Hg more than the control diet. This may not seem like much, but a systolic drop of just 5 mm Hg can cut your risk of suffering a stroke by an astounding 34 percent and the risk of a heart attack by 21 percent.[6]

Where's the Calcium?

Getting in 1,200 mg of calcium from foods is easier than you think. Take a look at the list of calcium power foods on pages 137–138 (or the Minerals Pocket Charts in Appendix 6) and get out your calculator. Your best bet is to go for the richest source of calcium out there, plain nonfat yogurt, and eat at least 2 cups a day. Eating 2 cups of plain nonfat yogurt, plus 1 cup of edamame and 1 cup of quinoa somewhere in your day easily puts you over the top.

Calcium Power Foods

Food	Serving Size	Calcium (mg)
Yogurt, nonfat	1 C	450
Yogurt, low-fat	1 C	415
Soy milk, calcium fortified	1 C	368
Collard greens, cooked	1 C	357
Sardines, canned, with bones	3.75 oz	351
Ricotta cheese, part skim	½ C	334
Milk, skim	1 C	306
Edamame	1 C	261
Tofu	½ C	253
Swiss cheese	1 oz	212
Salmon, canned, with bones	3 oz	188
Bok choy, steamed	1 C	158
Yogurt, Greek, nonfat	1 C	151
Feta cheese	1 oz	140
Blackstrap molasses	1 Tb	137
Navy beans, cooked	1 C	130
Black beans, cooked	1 C	120
Turnip greens, cooked	½ C	100
Quinoa, cooked	1 C	100
Kale, boiled	1 C	94
Almond butter	2 Tb	86
Celery, chopped	2 C	81
Pinto beans, cooked	1 C	80
Soy milk	1 C	80
Almonds, raw	24 nuts	75
Papaya	1 medium	73
Orange juice, freshly squeezed	1 C	72
Parmesan cheese	1 Tb	69
Cottage cheese, low-fat	½ C	69

Food	Serving Size	Calcium (mg)
Tahini	1 Tb	64
Herring	3 oz	63
Broccoli, cooked	1 C	62
Thyme, dried	1 Tb	57
Sweet potato, baked	1 medium	55
Dill, dried	1 Tb	53
Orange	1 medium	52
Chickpeas, cooked	½ C	40
Flaxseeds	1 Tb	26
Oregano, dried	1 Tb	21
Red pepper, chopped	1 C	10

GOING GREEK: NOT THE BEST CHOICE

Can you "go Greek" for your yogurt of choice? It tastes creamier and yummier than the conventional plain kind, and it packs in much more protein per ounce. But as blood pressure "medicine," Greek-style plain yogurt simply does not stack up against its non-Greek counterpart.

Here is a closer look at how two popular supermarket-ready yogurts compare, nutrition-wise:

	Fat-free plain yogurt (8-ounce container)	Fat-free plain Greek yogurt (6-ounce container)
Calories	100	100
Protein (g)	11	18
Sodium (mg)	150	80
Calcium (mg)	400	200
Potassium (mg)	510	250

You can see that to reach your daily goal of 1,200 mg of calcium (and 4,700 mg of potassium), choosing the conventional yogurt is your best bet—you get a bigger bang for your bite.

No matter which style you choose, it is important to opt for the plain nonfat varieties. Most of the flavored varieties simply have far too much added sugar. But don't despair—just because you buy it plain doesn't mean you have to eat it plain! Perhaps add some Splenda or even a touch of honey or molasses and save a bundle on the calories—another goal in the Blood Pressure Down plan.

BONING UP ON CALCIUM SCIENCE

Calcium-Rich Foods or Supplements: Which Is Best?

The science is in: adults who eat 1,000 to 1,500 mg of calcium per day reduce their risk of developing high blood pressure.[7] So what's better, taking a supplement or eating calcium from foods? Years ago, a highly comprehensive meta-analysis found that a diet high in calcium had *twice* the blood-pressure-lowering effect as calcium supplements.[8]

POWER DOWN YOUR PRESSURE: EAT FLAXSEEDS!

We know that flaxseeds are magnesium *and* calcium power foods— and now cutting-edge research out of Cuba, presented at the American Heart Association's 2012 Scientific Sessions, proves the blood-pressure-plummeting power of adding ground flaxseeds to your day. In a double-blind, placebo-controlled study called "**FLAX-PAD**," researchers at the University Hospital, Holguin, Cuba, added approximately four tablespoons of ground flaxseeds per day, containing a massive six grams of ALA, to the diets of patients with high blood pressure (many of the study participants also had concomitant peripheral artery disease). At the end of six months, the patients who ate the flaxseeds reduced their blood pressure by a remarkable 10 mm Hg systolic and 7 mm Hg diastolic, compared to those receiving a placebo. Those patients who also had peripheral artery disease achieved an even greater reduction in systolic blood pressure: a phenomenal 15 mm Hg!

The authors concluded that flaxseeds have a similar blood-pressure-lowering effect to prescription medication and surmised that the triple heart health package in flaxseeds—ALA omega-3 fat, lignan (a healthy hormone-like plant substance), and fiber—have a powerful synergistic effect on your arteries.

Source: American Heart Association *2012 Scientific Sessions Abstract 12080* (Hall A-12). Flaxseed may lower blood pressure in hypertension; http://newsroom.heart.org/pr/aha/monday-news-tips-november-5–2012–239565.aspx

That's not to say that calcium supplements are worthless. Two meta-analyses of numerous clinical trials of people with high (and normal) blood pressure showed that ingesting calcium supplements (400–2,000 mg/day) had a modest blood-pressure-lowering effect: almost 2 mm Hg systolic (top) and 0.2 mm Hg diastolic (bottom), respectively.[9,10] A more recent meta-analysis of forty studies involving more than twenty-five hundred subjects in the Netherlands also confirmed a small but statistically significant drop in blood pressure among people taking calcium supplements.[11] Those people taking an average of 1,200 mg of calcium a day lowered systolic pressure by 1.9 mm Hg along with a 1.0 mm Hg drop in diastolic. (The supplement worked better for people who typically ate low amounts of calcium; in that group, systolic blood pressure dropped by 2.6 mm Hg and diastolic by 1.3 mm Hg.)

These small drops stand in stark contrast to the results of studies involving people consuming low-fat, calcium-rich dairy foods. For example, an eight-week randomized clinical trial involving thirty-five healthy but overweight prehypertensive men and women saw great blood-pressure-lowering results from consuming low-fat milk or yogurt. This study followed a crossover design, meaning that the subjects were both the experimental group and the control group—they ate a control diet for eight weeks, followed by an additional eight weeks of the experimental diet (separated by a

GOT MILK?

Dairy foods are by far the leading source of calcium in the American diet. Does it matter what kind you eat? A systematic review of nearly forty-five thousand people examined the association between dairy foods and the development of high blood pressure and found that people consuming low-fat fluid dairy products (such as yogurt and milk) had the greatest reduction in risk of high blood pressure—16 percent—whereas consuming high-fat sources of dairy (such as cheese or ice cream) had no blood pressure benefit. The researchers think that the saturated fat, extra calories, and other inflammatory components in full-fat dairy negate the healthful blood-pressure-lowering effects.

Source: Ralston RA, Lee JH, Truby H, et al. A systematic review and meta-analysis of elevated blood pressure and consumption of dairy foods. *J Hum Hypertens* 2012;26:3–13.

two-week washout period). The only difference between the two diets was the amount of calcium from dairy foods (1,550 mg/day in the calcium diet, versus 931 mg/day in the control diet). The results? Following the calcium diet, systolic blood pressure was lowered by 2.9 mm Hg.[12]

As you know, participants in the original DASH diet combination group had similar blood-pressure-lowering results. The group eating an average of 1,265 mg of calcium a day through foods reduced their systolic pressure by 2.7 mm Hg and their diastolic pressure by 1.9 mm more than the fruits-and-vegetables-only group.[13] Clearly, eating calcium-containing foods rather than popping calcium pills is your best bet for lowering your millimeters of mercury through dietary changes.

Do Calcium Supplements Increase Heart Attack Risk?

Millions of Americans, especially postmenopausal women, take calcium supplements to prevent fractures and strengthen their bones against osteoporosis. Recent disturbing headlines have suggested that taking calcium supplements may actually increase the risk of having a heart attack. This claim stems from the highly controversial 2010 meta-analysis of data from the Women's Health Initiative (WHI), a fifteen-year multimillion-dollar project that pooled results from eleven studies that tracked nearly twelve thousand women.[14] Women taking an average of 1,000 mg of calcium a day were found to have a 27 percent higher risk of having a heart attack than those not taking supplements. The figures were alarming, but the results were immediately criticized by the scientific community. The main flaw in the study was that the analysis involved women taking calcium supplements alone, not calcium plus vitamin D—the more commonly recommended regimen. A reanalysis of the WHI data by the same authors found that the increased risk occurred among women who had never taken calcium supplements before and abruptly began the regimen of high-dose calcium supplementation.[15] The authors speculated that the rapid elevation of blood calcium levels contributed to the development of heart disease. They suggested obtaining calcium from food sources, from which the mineral is absorbed much more slowly.

A more recent large-scale study, in which German investigators examined data from nearly twenty-four thousand subjects, continues to question the safety of popping calcium pills.[16] The researchers found that those who took vitamin and mineral supplements (including calcium) on a regular basis were 86 percent more likely to have a heart attack than those not taking supplements. The risk increased further among those taking only calcium supplements—this group was twice as likely to have a heart attack compared to those who don't use supplements.

The takeaway message here? Large-scale, association-type studies like this don't allow us to deduce that calcium supplements *cause* heart attacks. Most scientists agree that there is not enough data to support a real link between supplemental calcium and heart

VITAMIN D WITH YOUR YOGURT, ANYONE?

It is best to buy a yogurt fortified with vitamin D, which enhances calcium absorption. Why do you need D with your calcium? A recent study showed that diabetics who ate vitamin-D-enriched yogurt every day significantly reduced markers of inflammation, thereby reducing heart disease risk. The problem is that most yogurts on the market are not fortified with vitamin D (they are not required by law to be). If you can't find a fortified nonfat yogurt, I recommend that you take a daily vitamin D supplement (see Chapter Twelve).

Sources: Calvo MS, Whiting SJ, Barton CN. Vitamin D fortification in the United States and Canada: current status and data needs. *Am J Clin Nutr* 2004;80(6 Suppl):1710S-1716S; Neyestani TR, Nikooyeh B, Alavi-Majd H, et al. Improvement of vitamin D status via daily intake of fortified yogurt drink either with or without extra calcium ameliorates systemic inflammatory biomarkers, including adpokines, in the subjects with type 2 diabetes. *J Clin Endocrinol Metab* 2012 June. DOI:10.1210/jc.2011–3465.

attacks. Therefore, if you are a postmenopausal woman, it is best to discuss supplementation with your doctor—there is no question that supplementation with calcium plus vitamin D is effective in reducing bone fractures in postmenopausal women. For everyone else, it is ideal to aim for eating your calcium in the form of food rather than supplements.

One arm of the WHI supports the advice to consume calcium- and vitamin-D-rich foods as opposed to supplements. In this sub-sample of the WHI, scientists conducted a randomized trial of more than thirty-six thousand healthy postmenopausal women given supplemental calcium (1,000 mg) plus vitamin D_3 (400 international units, or IU) daily. Over a seven-year period, the supplements did not reduce blood pressure or reduce the risk of developing prehypertension or full-blown hypertension.[17]

As another large-scale observational study confirms, eating your calcium is your best bet for blood pressure control. The Women's

Health Study (WHS) followed 28,886 middle-aged and older women for ten years and found that the higher a woman's intake of low-fat dairy products, calcium, and vitamin D from food, the lower her risk of developing high blood pressure.[18]

What Is It in Calcium-Rich Foods That Lowers Blood Pressure?

We know that calcium in and of itself has a small blood-pressure-lowering effect. However, the association between eating high-calcium, low-fat dairy products and a reduction in blood pressure is much stronger, suggesting that there's something else in dairy foods that helps with blood pressure control. So find out how calcium and dairy products work together to rein in those millimeters of mercury.

Method of attack #1: When you don't have enough calcium in your diet, something called a "calcium leak" occurs in your kidneys. This means that the kidneys excrete more calcium in the urine, disturbing the balance of mineral metabolism involved in blood pressure regulation. Consuming enough calcium (and potassium) in the diet "fixes" the leak, conserving minerals and normalizing blood pressure.[19]

Method of attack #2: Dairy products contain a milk-derived protein that has a blood-pressure-lowering effect in prehypertensive people, as well as those with diagnosed high blood pressure.[20] This protein works like a natural ACE inhibitor, interfering with the conversion of angiotensin I into angiotensin II, the highly potent blood vessel constrictor that drives blood pressure up, fast. Lessen the amount of angiotensin II, and you automatically lower your pressure.

Method of attack #3: Eating yogurt can help keep your weight in check—another goal of the Blood Pressure Down plan. A Harvard study published in the prestigious *New England Journal of Medicine* found that people tended to lose nearly a pound every four years just by adding a yogurt to their day.[21]

CALCIUM CAVEATS

Calcium supplements can interfere with certain prescription medications, so you may want to think twice before turning to supplements to get your calcium. For example, if you are taking a thiazide diuretic or "water pill" (such as hydrochlorothiazide), then you need to be careful how much calcium you take in supplement form. Taking 1,500 mg or more of calcium with thiazide diuretics can result in milk-alkali syndrome, a serious condition that is particularly dangerous for your kidneys.

If you are eating the prescribed amount of calcium from foods, there is no need to take extra in the form of a supplement. If you do choose to take a calcium supplement while taking prescription medications, make sure to talk to your doctor about potential drug-nutrient interactions, and have your calcium levels checked frequently. Remember, the right amount of calcium is healthful (as we learned in the previous chapter), whereas too much is harmful.

You should also get your vitamin D level checked. The normal range is 30.0 to 74.0 nanograms per milliliter (ng/mL). If yours is lower than that, talk to your doctor; I suggest you take a daily supplement of vitamin D_3, 1,000–2,000 IU, under your doctor's supervision. As we've learned, vitamin D is crucial for helping your body absorb calcium.

FILLING THE PRESCRIPTION

Eating two fat-free yogurts, a 10-ounce bag of fresh spinach (which shrinks into a minuscule portion when cooked), two kiwis, and a handful of soy nuts will easily get you to your daily calcium goal. If any of these foods are not your cup of tea, then mix and match from the list of calcium power foods or from the Minerals Pocket Charts in Appendix 6.

FIVE TIPS FOR GETTING YOGURT INTO YOUR DAY

You just can't beat a cup of plain fat-free yogurt a day to make a huge dent in your calcium prescription for relatively few calories. It can have as much as 400 mg of calcium (plus tons of other vitamins and minerals), all for just about 100 calories. Considering that a cup of plain nonfat yogurt is the top source of calcium, you may want to consider eating yogurt as your go-to snack of choice. Here are some examples of the delicious versatility of yogurt:

1. Mix it with seasonings such as garlic, dill, and parsley and use as a dip for veggies.
2. Swirl in some low-sugar fruit preserves and use as a dip for fresh fruit.
3. Plop some yogurt on your morning bowl of oatmeal, add a tablespoon or two of ground flaxseeds and fresh berries, and you have a quick and healthy fiber-packed breakfast.
4. Use fat-free yogurt in place of water in baked goods and pancakes. You will be surprised at how this simple swap can add both taste and nutrition to your recipes.
5. For a tasty and super-nutritious treat, try what I call "pumpkin pie yogurt." Add a few tablespoons of solid-pack plain pumpkin (and get another potassium boost too!) to an 8-ounce container of yogurt, along with half a teaspoon or so of pumpkin pie spice and two packets of Splenda Essentials with fiber. Mix it all up; then top with fat-free whipped topping and some finely diced walnuts . . . yum!

As you can see, you can lower your blood pressure naturally by simply eating a few foods that are affordable and readily available at your local supermarket. You knew that this dietary move could strengthen your bones, but now you know that calcium is also a key player in your blood-pressure-lowering "mineral diet." Pay close attention to reaching your daily calcium goal of at least

1,200 mg of calcium from foods, and you will be packing a powerful blood-pressure-lowering daily dietary punch.

So, you have learned that losing just a few pounds, shaking the salt habit, and filling your plate with foods rich in potassium, magnesium, and calcium are mighty potent lifestyle steps for getting your pressure where you need it to be. Next we're going to round out your plate with a perfect source of healthy plant protein. Let's address the blood-pressure-lowering joy of eating soy.

Step 6: Eat Soy

Eat 25 g of Soy Protein in Place of Animal Protein Every Day

Eat more plant protein and less animal protein—that's the mantra for those who truly want to lower their blood pressure naturally. Americans who are striving to stay healthy and pare down those millimeters of mercury should open their minds (and mouths) to the idea of adding soy to their daily diet. Soy is a high-quality plant protein, meaning it provides all the essential amino acids required in the human diet, and unlike animal protein, it contains zero cholesterol and only a minute amount of artery-clogging saturated fat. What's more, eating soy protein has been proven to lower blood pressure, whereas eating animal protein—specifically red and processed meats—increases blood pressure.[1] Just how hard is it to get 25 grams of soy protein into your day? As easy as adding 12 ounces of soy milk to your morning bowl of oatmeal and snacking on a quarter cup of dry-roasted, unsalted soy nuts.

MAKING THE SWITCH

Why substitute tofu for beef jerky? There are many reasons why swapping plant protein for red meat and processed meats is a wise nutrition move. An excessive intake of both red and processed meat in your diet contributes to high blood pressure—and can cut your life short. In fact, a large-scale study recently published in the *Archives of Internal Medicine,* in which scientists followed more than a hundred thousand men and women for twenty years, found that eating both processed and unprocessed red meat was associated with an increased risk of premature death from cancer and cardiovascular diseases.[2] Here's why:

- Red meat, such as hamburgers and steak, is a major source of a kind of iron called heme iron. Heme iron is highly bioavailable, meaning your body absorbs it quickly and easily. Nonheme iron, which is found in vegetable proteins, is less readily available to the body. Too much iron causes oxidative injury to the inner lining of the blood vessels and has also been linked with inflammation—two harmful processes that must be reversed to lower blood pressure and prevent heart disease and stroke. (But for those of us at risk for iron deficiency, including vegetarians, teenage girls, women of childbearing age, pregnant women, and the elderly, heme iron is the better choice—though with a little planning, vegetarians can easily meet their iron requirements, too.)

- As you know from Chapter Five, processed red meats are overloaded with sodium. Eat just one hot dog and you've consumed almost half of your daily sodium allowance—and that's without the condiments or roll!

- Red meats are high in saturated fat and dietary cholesterol. (The hot dog we just talked about contains 5 grams of artery-clogging saturated fat!) This raises the amount of "bad" LDL cholesterol in your blood and thus increases your risk for heart attack and stroke.

- Red meat, especially processed meat, contains nitrates and other carcinogens that are formed during cooking.
- Red meat is higher in calories compared to skinless poultry, fish, or vegetable sources of protein. A higher calorie intake contributes to the obesity epidemic.

More Plants, Less Animals = A Leaner, Lighter, Low-Pressure You

Substituting plant protein for animal protein is a perfect diet strategy that will help you lose both millimeters of mercury *and* pounds. The fact is that vegetarians as a group have lower blood pressure

SOY NUTS: A PROVEN BLOOD-PRESSURE-LOWERING SNACK

The results are in: just half a cup a day of roasted soybeans (known as "soy nuts," though soybeans are legumes, not true nuts) cuts blood pressure as much as medication! According to an eight-week randomized controlled clinical trial of sixty postmenopausal women, published in the *Archives of Internal Medicine*, a daily ½-cup serving of dry-roasted, salt-free soy nuts (which provides 25 grams of soy protein and 101 mg of isoflavones, the blood-pressure-lowering substance in soy) reduced systolic blood pressure by a whopping 10 percent and diastolic blood pressure by 7 percent in women with diagnosed high blood pressure, and by 5 percent and 3 percent in women with normal blood pressure. The blood-pressure-lowering effect of soy, according to the researchers, was comparable to the effects of prescription medication.

Dry-roasted, unsalted soy nuts can't be beat for a low-calorie, tasty, blood-pressure-lowering snack. They are exceptionally high in protein, practically sodium free, and have a low glycemic index. This makes them a perfect snack—they are filling, don't give your blood sugar level a jolt, and contribute to lasting energy.

Source: Welty FK, Lee KS, Lew N, Zhou J-R. Effect of soy nuts on blood pressure and lipid levels in hypertensive, prehypertensive, and normotensive postmenopausal women. *Arch Intern Med* 2007;167:1060–1067.

and are leaner and lighter than meat eaters[3]—reason enough to choose beans over beef. But it's not just about weight. Eating lower on the food chain clearly affects blood pressure. A large study of nearly five thousand middle-aged people in four countries, published in the prestigious *Archives of Internal Medicine,* documented that people with a high intake of vegetable protein and a low intake of animal protein have lower blood pressure (4.15 mm Hg lower systolic pressure and 2.15 mm Hg lower diastolic) compared to people who consume a diet high in animal protein and low in vegetable protein.[4]

SOY SCIENCE

Just how do we know that eating soy foods lowers blood pressure? There is an ever-growing body of solid scientific evidence that supports the blood-pressure-friendly effect of eating soy foods. One great example is the Shanghai Women's Health Study, a large analysis of nearly fifty thousand healthy middle-aged and elderly Chinese women. This is a population that routinely eats soy as a staple in their diet. When scientists took a close look at the women's health, an interesting phenomenon surfaced: the higher the soy food intake, the lower both systolic and diastolic blood pressure numbers were, particularly among the older women. The systolic pressure was 4.9 mm Hg lower and the diastolic 2.2 mm Hg lower in elderly women who consumed more than 25 grams of soy protein a day compared to those consuming less than 2.5 grams a day.[5] As you can see, this small but mighty bean has a distinct beneficial effect on blood pressure numbers.

Clinical Trials Prove Soy Slashes Blood Pressure Numbers

Even if you've never incorporated soy into your diet before, if you start to add some soy to your day now, you will see blood-pressure-lowering benefits. Numerous randomized clinical

GOT HIGH BLOOD PRESSURE? SOY GETS IT DOWN!

Hot off the presses is a meta-analysis of the effect of soy isoflavones on blood pressure. In the study, published in the journal *Nutrition, Metabolism and Cardiovascular Diseases*, Chinese scientists analyzed data from eleven randomized, double-blind, placebo-controlled clinical trials (the gold standard of research proving cause and effect). The dosage of soy isoflavones in the studies ranged from 65 to 153 mg/day. The results? For those people with diagnosed high blood pressure, switching over to soy food lowered their systolic blood pressure 6 mm Hg and diastolic pressure 3 mm Hg.

Source: Liu XX, Li SH, Chen JZ, et al. Effect of soy isoflavones on blood pressure: A meta-analysis of randomized controlled trials. *Nutrition, Metabolism & Cardiovascular Diseases* 2012;22:463–470.

trials have shown that even short-term soy intake significantly reduces both systolic and diastolic blood pressure,[6,7,8,9] with substantially greater reductions noted in people with high blood pressure compared to subjects with normal blood pressure at baseline.[10] Case in point: a well-designed randomized clinical trial out of China in which researchers randomly assigned more than three hundred men and women (ages thirty-five to sixty-four) with prehypertension or stage 1 high blood pressure to either 40 grams of soy protein (76 mg of isoflavones) per day or a placebo for twelve weeks.[11] The soy protein group saw systolic and diastolic blood pressure reductions of 7.14 mm Hg and 4.72 mm Hg (for people with high blood pressure) and 2.49 mm Hg and 1.32 mm Hg (for those with prehypertension).

Even meat-loving Scots benefited from replacing some animal protein with soy protein! In a study of the effect of soy intake on cardiovascular disease risk factors, researchers recruited 156 middle-aged men with high blood pressure living on the Isles of

Lewis and Harris (in the northwest of Scotland). For five weeks, the men were randomly assigned to a diet containing either 20 grams of soy protein (80 mg of isoflavones) or a control diet. Following the intervention period, both groups of men maintained the same starting body weight. But the soy group showed an astounding drop in blood pressure: 11 mm Hg systolic and 5 mm Hg diastolic, compared to no change in the control group.[12] Clearly, the blood pressure benefits of soy are not just about weight loss.

WHY EAT SOY?

Eating soy is associated with a variety of health benefits. This is because, like all beans, soybeans contain all sorts of health-promoting ingredients: dietary fiber, B vitamins (including the heart-healthy folic acid), calcium, iron, phytochemicals (which protect against a host of diseases), and essential omega-3 fats. The composition of a soybean is 38 percent protein, 30 percent carbohydrate, 20 percent fat (mostly polyunsaturated), and the rest moisture. The protein found in soybeans is unique among plant proteins: unlike other beans, soy is a high-quality protein, meaning it provides all the essential amino acids required in the human diet. But unlike animal protein, it contains zero cholesterol and only a tiny amount of saturated fat.

Feast on Flavonoids to Cut Pressure and Live Longer

The next time you are faced with a choice between meatless chili brimming with beans and hearty vegetables and the cheesy meat-filled traditional style, go for the vegetarian version. The science is clear: people who eat lots of plant foods and less animal foods have lower blood pressure. Not only do the plant foods provide you with a natural source of our trio of blood-pressure-lowering mineral superstars (potassium, magnesium, and calcium), they also house fiber as well as another star player in the Blood Pressure Down plan: flavonoids.

What are flavonoids, you may ask? Flavonoids are a calorie-free bioactive plant chemical with wonderfully potent anti-inflammatory effects. Humans cannot synthesize flavonoids, so we must eat them in our diet. Flavonoids are found in a range of plant-based foods, including spinach, kale, nuts, dark chocolate, red wine, and soy. There are numerous classes of flavonoids, but five are specifically linked to a host of health benefits: anthocyanins, flavan-3-ols, flavones, procyanidins, and isoflavones. Soy is the only commonly eaten food that contains a biologically relevant concentration of the class of flavonoids known as isoflavones. (And if you really want to know, the two most famous isoflavones go by the chemical names genistein and diadzein.)

What do scientists have to say about flavonoids? Eating lots of them can protect you from ever developing high blood pressure in the first place. A Japanese study followed 745 men and women (without high blood pressure) for four years and found that those with the highest flavonoid intake had a 60 percent reduced risk of developing high blood pressure.[13] Here on our home turf, research shows that a high intake of flavonoids not only cuts blood pressure but can also cut your risk of dying prematurely. A recent study of the dietary habits of nearly a hundred thousand older American men and women, published in the *American Journal of Clinical Nutrition*, found that individuals consuming a high amount of flavonoids (twenty servings of fruit and twenty-four servings of vegetables per week) had an 18 percent lower risk of dying from cardiovascular problems than men and women with a low intake of flavonoids.[14]

SOY SAFETY

Soy is a safe and wholesome food that has been a staple protein source of East Asian populations for centuries. In fact, Chinese people have eaten it for at least five thousand years, and the Japanese for a thousand years. There are actually two types of soy foods: unfermented and fermented. Tofu, soy milk, and edamame (pronounced "ay-duh-MAH-may") are examples of unfermented soy foods. Examples of fermented soy foods include natto (a popular Japanese delicacy made from soybeans that have been soaked and fermented to a sticky, stringy consistency), miso (not the best choice due to the outrageous sodium content), and tempeh. You may have heard rumors that only fermented soy foods are healthful, but there is little scientific proof that this is true. In fact, most of the studies proving the health benefits of soy have used unfermented soy products such as soy milk or soy nuts in the research.

Worried About a Possible Link Between Soy and Breast Cancer?

You might have read headlines that eating soy is linked to developing breast cancer. Let's take a look at the science. Human estrogens play a key role in promoting the growth of estrogen-dependent breast cancer tumors (the most common type). In fact, more than 80 percent of breast cancer tumors in women over forty-five are activated by the human hormone estrogen via proteins called estrogen receptors. Isoflavones, found in soy, are classified as a phytoestrogen, or plant estrogen, because they are capable of binding to estrogen receptors on cell walls. However, plant estrogens bind to and activate a set of estrogen receptors that is separate from those for the human hormone estrogen. The result is very weak estrogenic effects, meaning soy does not fuel breast cancer tumor growth.

The scientific evidence is clear: soy foods are safe and do not cause breast cancer. In fact, just the opposite is true: eating soy food protects you against developing breast cancer. You should know that Asian women consume an average of 25 to 50 mg of isoflavones per day (more than ten times what the average Western woman consumes) and have just one-fifth the rate of breast cancer.[15] I suggest that you aim for eating 25 grams of soy protein a day from whole foods. Each gram will provide you with approximately 3.5 mg of isoflavones, making it a cinch to reach another of your Blood Pressure Down goals: over 50 mg isoflavones per day. Remember, a diet high in whole, unprocessed soy foods has a long history of safety and health-related benefits. (It is the isolated soy supplements that you should be wary of.)

If you have already been diagnosed with breast cancer, studies have shown that soy can improve your prognosis, reducing your risk of death and disease recurrence.[16,17] The American Cancer Society states that breast cancer survivors can consume soy foods in their diets—though it cautions against more concentrated sources of soy, such as pills or powders. (This is because the science has proven the safety of consuming soy food, whereas the safety of concentrated sources of soy has not been adequately researched.)

Real Men Eat Soy

Men concerned about any potential feminizing effect of soy can also rest assured that soy intake does not decrease testosterone levels or increase estrogen levels.[18,19] A recent meta-analysis out of the University of Minnesota found that soy intake does not affect sex hormone concentrations in men, regardless of age.[20] Clinical studies have also clarified that soy isoflavone consumption does not adversely affect sperm concentration, count, or motility.[21,22]

Not All Soy Is Good

There are four whole foods that are best for obtaining your soy prescription: soy milk, soybeans (edamame or soy nuts), tofu, and tempeh. Unfortunately, reaching for the salad dressing made with soybean oil won't help you reap the phenomenal health benefits of soy foods. Americans use massive quantities of soybean oil, a cheap source of fat that is ubiquitous in the world of processed foods. But only soy foods that contain soy protein confer substantial health benefits. You can and should avoid soybean oil (and replace it with

---

SOY MILK: IT DOES A BLOOD VESSEL GOOD

In a three-month randomized clinical study of forty men and women with mild to moderate high blood pressure, scientists found that simply adding in four 8-ounce cups a day of soy milk lowered systolic pressure by a spectacular 18.4 mm Hg and diastolic by 15.9 mm Hg (compared to 1.4 to 3.7 mm Hg reduction in the group drinking cow's milk).

Source: Rivas M, Garay RP, Escanero JF, et al. Soy milk lowers blood pressure in men and women with mild to moderate essential hypertension. *J Nutr* 2002;132:1900–1902.

---

heart-healthier oils such as extra-virgin olive oil and canola oil) by checking for it on food labels, under various names such as "vegetable oil" or "hydrolyzed soybean oil."

Soy sauce is another food that has soy in its name but does *not* count toward your daily soy prescription. Far from a healthful soy protein, soy sauce contains an enormous amount of sodium and only a minimal amount of health-promoting soy ingredients.

What Exactly Is in Soybeans That Lowers Blood Pressure?

The heart-healthy benefits of soy are well documented and are attributed to several actions involving phytoestrogens, amino acids, and antioxidants. Here are the main mechanisms through which plant protein, and soy in particular, lower your blood pressure.

Method of attack #1: As you know, an important feature of a healthy artery is adequate production of the key blood vessel relaxation chemical nitric oxide by the cells lining the inner arterial wall. In people with elevated blood pressure, the production of nitric oxide is compromised and the arteries cannot dilate as well in response to the nitric oxide that is synthesized. The isoflavones in soy enhance the activity of the enzyme responsible for the production of nitric oxide. Soy isoflavones therefore play a role in relaxing the arteries—and easing the pressure.[23,24]

Method of attack #2: Vegetable protein, specifically soy protein, has a high concentration of the amino acid arginine. Some scientists believe soy's arginine content explains soy's substantial blood pressure benefits.[25] Arginine is extremely healthful for the arteries because it is a building block that the body uses to make nitric oxide. You already know that nitric oxide lowers blood pressure. Nitric oxide also makes the blood less sticky, which helps to prevent the formation of a lethal blood clot that can lead to a heart attack or stroke.

Method of attack #3: Soy not only is good for the arteries but also improves the health of your kidneys, decreases blood sugar levels, and makes muscles more sensitive to insulin—making you less likely to develop insulin resistance, which (as you learned in Chapter Two) is a major risk factor for hypertension.[26]

Method of attack #4: People with high blood pressure and vascular disease also tend to have endothelial dysfunction, meaning their arterial cells are unable to fight effectively against inflammation, blood clots, and oxidative stress.[27] Soy protein intake has been shown to have a beneficial anti-inflammatory effect on the endothelium, especially in people with diagnosed high blood pressure, who usually have some degree of inflammation. How do we know that soy soothes the flames burning within the arterial walls? A group of Harvard researchers answered this question in a study of sixty postmenopausal women with high blood pressure and associated inflammation in the arteries, who were fed a half cup of soy nuts a day (25 grams of soy protein and 101 mg of isoflavones) for 8 weeks. Scientists documented a significant decline in a blood marker of inflammation in the arteries of women with previously diagnosed high blood pressure on the soy diet, compared to no change in women on the control diet.[28]

Method of attack #5: By adding soy protein to your diet, you tend to eliminate some red meat, which is often loaded with saturated fat and cholesterol. Cut your saturated fat and cholesterol intake, and you'll automatically lower your "bad" LDL cholesterol and decrease your risk for a heart attack or stroke. What's more, replacing high-calorie animal protein with much-lower-calorie soy protein will significantly drop your calorie intake, a great strategy for helping you lose those five pounds and cut your blood pressure down to size.

SOY CAUTION

Soy does tend to be a highly allergenic food, particularly in children. If you're sensitive to soy, of course avoid eating soy products. Soy may also cause problems with thyroid function—some scientific evidence even suggests a link between soy consumption and goiter. But the consensus is that in healthy individuals, soy consumption does not adversely affect thyroid function. If you've been diagnosed with thyroid dysfunction, talk to your doctor and be cautious about consuming soy products.

Soy foods can also be high in fat and calories. A cup of full-fat soy milk contains 125 calories and 5 grams of fat. That's 40 more calories and 5 more grams of fat than a glass of fat-free soy milk. Your best bet is to buy the "light," unsweetened soy milk varieties; you will still get the soy protein and isoflavones, only with fewer calories in the bargain. Soy nuts are a tasty way to add soy into your day—but keep in mind that they are high in calories. Eat too many and you'll pay at the scale. Stick to 1 ounce (about ¼ cup) for a healthy snack.

FILLING THE PRESCRIPTION

Americans should include soy foods in their diet on a daily basis, to the tune of 20–25 grams of soy protein per day, which amounts to three or four servings of soy—and adds up to 100 mg of artery-friendly isoflavones. This is a practical, inexpensive, and safe way to reduce blood pressure. Eating this amount will not harm you—it will heal your arteries and help you to prevent and even treat heart disease. Try to get your soy from the whole foods listed below and not from the salt-laden processed types (check the labels of the plethora of soy products on the freezer shelf and you will see what I mean). One of the easiest ways to get your soy is to simply replace cow's milk with light, unsweetened soy milk. Another tasty option is edamame, which you can order at Japanese restaurants (steamed and without salt), or purchase frozen at your local health food store or grocery store and cook at home in your microwave.

Soy Food	Serving Size and Calories	Soy Protein Content
Tempeh	½ C (4 oz) (200 cal)	19 g
Tofu (firm)	½ C (4 oz) (70 cal)	13–20 g
Edamame	½ C (40 cal)	11 g
Soy nuts (unsalted, dry roasted)	¼ C (250 cal)	10–15 g
Plain soy milk	8 oz (125 cal)	6 g
Light soy milk	8 oz (70 cal)	6 g
Soy nut butter	2 Tb (170 cal)	8 g
Soy flour	¼ C (90 cal)	7 g

Here are six easy ways to add soy protein to your daily diet:

1. Substitute soy milk for cow's milk. Use it in shakes, on cereal, in baking, in puddings, and just about anywhere else that you would typically use cow's milk.
2. Eat a bowl of steamed and unsalted edamame.
3. Snack on unsalted, dry-roasted soy nuts. Try tossing some in your salad for added crunch or even in your daily

yogurt. They're incredibly portable—you can stash a plastic bag of soy nuts almost anywhere. Most important, their hearty flavor makes them a delicious snack that you'll surely enjoy eating.

4. Learn to cook with tofu (I like the extra-firm style). It is very versatile and takes on the flavor of whatever you cook it with. You can stir-fry it, blend it into smoothies, add it to soups, puree it into dips and spreads, or eat it in salads.

5. Try tempeh, a textured soy product with a firmer and chewier texture than tofu. Like tofu, it absorbs the flavors around it, making it another versatile plant protein for cooking. Try stir-frying, baking, or even grilling tempeh.

6. Try a soy nut butter and banana sandwich (on whole-grain bread, of course!).

You have learned how powerful soy foods are in ameliorating dysfunctional arteries. Eat more plant foods and fewer animal foods and it will be just a matter of time before you reap the tremendous benefits for heart and blood vessel health. What's more, by getting in your daily exercise and eating plant protein in lieu of high-fat, high-calorie animal protein, you will pare down your waistline while you whittle away your millimeters of mercury. Getting your flavonoids from a variety of different foods every day is the Blood Pressure Down method that attacks vessel disease from multiple angles. Read on to learn about another fabulous source of natural plant flavonoids—deep, dark, sinfully delicious chocolate!

Step 7: Eat Dark Chocolate

 Eat 2 Tablespoons of Natural, Unsweetened Cocoa Powder or One or Two Squares of Dark Chocolate Every Day

Chocolate lovers rejoice! Believe it or not, this "forbidden food" is actually a magical blood-pressure-lowering medication. How do we know this? Take the indigenous Kuna Indian population of the San Blas Islands of Panama. They practically never get high blood pressure, nor is there any evidence that their blood pressure climbs with age. Yet when the Kuna Islanders relocate to urban areas of mainland Panama and change their dietary habits accordingly, their pressure shoots up with age and high blood pressure is common. Why the difference in disease rates between the indigenous Kuna and their urban counterparts? It certainly isn't genetics. The answer to this puzzle lies in their eating habits: indigenous Kuna consume enormous amounts of a superb blood-pressure-lowering food, cocoa—a whopping five cups every day![1]

CHOCOLATE: ANCIENT MEDICINE

Cacao—the small tropical tree whose seeds (which we call cacao beans) are fermented, then used to make powdered cocoa and chocolate—has a long history. Cultivation of cacao can be traced back thousands of years to the great Olmec settlements of Mesoamerica. Vessels for drinking chocolate dating from approximately A.D. 450 to 500 have been found at the burial sites of the ancient Maya nobility in Mexico and Central America. Both the Maya and the Aztec offered cacao as a gift to the gods, prompting Carl Linneaus, the Swedish botanist and father of modern taxonomy, to name the cacao tree *Theobroma cacao,* literally "food of the gods." For thousands of years, the fruits of the cacao tree have also been used as medicine to treat everything from depression and fatigue to a poor sex drive. Cocoa as a beverage came to Europe in the sixteenth century, brought back by the discoverers of the New World, and in the nineteenth century it became a luxury item. In Britain in the early 1800s, cocoa was transformed from primarily a beverage (without sugar) into the solid chocolate confections (with added sugar and milk) that so many of us worship today.[2]

Cocoa and Chocolate Are Two Different Things

Although it is tempting to put chocolate and cocoa into the same health category, they mean quite different things. After harvest, the seeds from the cacao tree are fermented, dried, cleaned, and roasted. Then the nibs (the "meat" of the cocoa bean, after the outer layer is removed) are ground into a thick, dark brown paste called chocolate liquor. Chocolate liquor consists of cocoa butter (fat) and cocoa solids (nonfat cocoa powder or finely ground cocoa beans). The fat in cocoa butter is mostly saturated (albeit one-third is stearic acid, a saturated fat that has a neutral effect on blood cholesterol level).[3] Cocoa solids are the nonfat, healthful component of the liquor.

Chocolate is a confection made of cocoa solids, cocoa butter, sugar, and sometimes milk, formed into a solid food product. With its high sugar and fat content, this form of your blood pressure medicine is certainly not a health food. Your best bet is to aim for

CHOCOLATE: THE NEW DIET FOOD

In a recent study published in the esteemed *Archives of Internal Medicine*, scientists analyzed the dietary habits of nearly a thousand healthy men and women ages twenty to eighty-five and found that frequent chocolate eaters had the lowest body weight (measured as body mass index). The San Diego–based researchers surmise that the catechins in chocolate may possess antioxidant properties that favorably influence metabolism.

Source: Golumb BA, Koperski S, White HL. Association between more frequent chocolate consumption and lower body mass index. *Arch Intern Med* 2012;172(6):519–521.

ingesting mostly the cocoa solids, which are low in calories and virtually fat-free.

All cocoa solids are high in flavonoids, a type of polyphenol antioxidant.[4] It's what happens during the processing that determines if the final chocolate product retains the healthful flavonoids. Because flavonoids are bitter, manufacturers may remove many of them from natural cocoa and add sugar and milk to enhance flavor—although certain chocolate manufacturers, such as Mars and Barry Callebaut, have developed proprietary methods of processing cocoa that retains the flavonoid content.

Dark chocolate—with a high content of nonfat cocoa solids—is now the new guilt-free superfood! What's the magic ingredient in dark chocolate that confers so many benefits? You guessed it—it's the flavonoids. And cocoa (that has not been heavily processed) contains *lots* of flavonoids. In fact, dark chocolate has such a highly concentrated amount of flavonoids that it beats out red wine.

Color is not everything, though. "Dutching" (or alkalization) of cocoa, for example, makes the chocolate taste milder but also removes almost all of the flavonoids.[5] Although Dutch cocoa is intensely dark in color, it's not the depth of the color that should alert you to the health benefits of the product. Instead, the important factor is the flavonoid content—which in Dutch cocoa has been severely depleted. (Note that the exact amount of flavonoids in commercial chocolate products is not publicly available yet, but it is likely that manufacturers will report those values in the not-too-distant future.)

There are many cocoa and chocolate products on the market today, so it's important to know which contain the greatest blood-pressure-lowering antioxidant power. Researchers at the Hershey Company analyzed the commercially available chocolate-containing products and found that the level of cocoa solids was the main factor in determining antioxidant activity. Predictably, the more cocoa solids were in a product, the better. Natural cocoa powders (ground cocoa solids) had the highest level of flavonoids, followed by unsweetened baking chocolates, dark chocolates, and

NEW STUDY: EPICATECHIN SLASHES BLOOD PRESSURE

A recent meta-analysis of randomized, controlled clinical trials showed that a daily treat of flavonoid-rich cocoa can have a huge blood-pressure-lowering effect. For this analysis, German researchers investigated the effects of one cocoa flavonoid in particular: epicatechin. Results showed that a daily intake of 25 mg of epicatechin (the amount in approximately 1 ounce of dark chocolate) cut systolic blood pressure by 4.1 mm Hg and diastolic by 2.0 mm Hg. The authors noted that epicatechin increases the level of nitric oxide, a potent vasodilator that relaxes the smooth muscle cells of the arteries, allowing the blood vessels to loosen and expand.

Source: Ellinger S, Reusch A, Stehle P, Helfrich H-P. Epicatechin ingested via cocoa products reduces blood pressure in humans: a nonlinear regression model with a Bayesian approach. *Am J Clin Nutr* 2012. DOI:10.3945/ajcn.111.029330.

semisweet chocolate baking chips. Milk chocolate and chocolate syrup contained the fewest flavonoids.[6] Do your blood vessels a favor—choose your chocolate wisely and opt for making your own sweet treats from flavonoid-packed natural unsweetened cocoa powder. Cocoa nibs are basically peeled, roasted, and crushed cacoa beans. As they are not highly processed and have no additives, cocoa nibs have a very intense bitter flavor. You may consider grinding the cocoa nibs and adding them to your coffee grounds for a blood-pressure-lowering morning cocktail.

FANTASTIC FLAVONOIDS

As you learned in the last chapter, flavonoids are one class of polyphenols, potent plant chemicals known for their spectacular antioxidant and anti-inflammatory actions. Flavonoids are calorie-free bioactive plant chemicals that are spectacular medicine for the arteries. There are several main subclasses of flavonoids, all characterized by a similar chemical structure. Soy, for example, contains large quantities of the isoflavone subclass of flavonoids. When it comes to chocolate, what is even more important than the concentration of flavonoids is the *type* of flavonoid subclass cocoa contains— flavan-3-ols (see Figure 10.1). This potent subclass, which does wonders for your arteries, makes up 99 percent of all the polyphenols found in cocoa and cocoa products. (For you science buffs, the substances that constitute the flavan-3-ol subclass of flavonoids are epicatechins, catechins, and procyanidins.)[7]

Not All Chocolate Is Created Equal

Keep in mind that it's the cocoa component of chocolate that contains the blood-pressure-lowering ingredient, flavonoids—so the higher the percentage of cocoa solids, the more flavonoids. More cocoa can sometimes mean less sugar and more bitterness, but it's best to choose dark chocolate that's highest in cocoa mass, even if you have to sacrifice some of the taste. Often, the front of

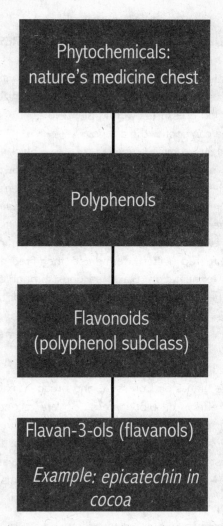

Figure 10.1 Chocolate contains an extraordinarily large concentration of the flavonoid subclass of polyphenols, the powerful subgroup called flavan-3-ols, or flavanols.

chocolate packages and sometimes the ingredients list indicate the percentage of cocoa solids (or cocoa mass) in the product such as 55 percent cocoa mass or 72 percent cocoa mass. Sample several different dark chocolate products until you find one that appeals to you. Watch out for imposters such as white chocolate, hot chocolate mixes, chocolate syrups, and milk chocolate bars, all of which are low in flavonoids.

TEA: THREE CUPS A DAY KEEPS HIGH BLOOD PRESSURE AWAY

Just like chocolate, tea is a plant food—and plants contain a plethora of phytochemicals that, when stacked together, maximize the strength of your daily blood-pressure-lowering plan. No doubt about it: a few daily cups of tea can soothe the arteries.

There are three main varieties of tea—black, oolong, and green—and all are derived from the tea plant known as *Camellia sinensis.* (Countless herbal infusions are informally referred to as "tea," but these are unrelated to real tea produced from *Camellia sinensis.*) Teas are classified based on how the leaves are processed. *Green* tea, the least processed of the three, is dried but not fermented. Oolong tea has been withered (wilted), fermented, then fired directly to prevent continued fermentation. Black tea goes through the most processing. Here the tea leaves have been fermented for a much longer period, a process that gives black tea its darker color and richer flavor. The predominant disease-fighting flavonoid in all forms of tea is the catechins.

Animal studies have shown that administration of green tea extract prevents high blood pressure and organ damage. And black tea's favorable effects on blood pressure were recently researched in humans. In a six-month randomized clinical trial of a hundred men and women, drinking three cups of black tea a day was found to lower systolic and diastolic numbers by 2–3 mm Hg. Just be sure not to add milk to your tea—the addition of milk completely blunts the favorable effect of tea on arterial function.

Sources: Antonello M, Montemurro D, Bolognesi M, et al. Prevention of hypertension, cardiovascular damage and endothelial dysfunction with green tea extracts. *Am J Hypertens* 2007;20:1321–1328; Hodgson JM, Puddey IB, Woodman RJ, et al. Effects of black tea on blood pressure: a randomized controlled trial. *Arch Intern Med* 2012;172(2):186–188; Lorenz M, Jochmann N, von Krosigk A, et al. Addition of milk prevents vascular protective effects of tea. *Am Heart J* 2007;28:219–223.

Because the cocoa solids contain the lion's share of the anti-oxidant polyphenols and the cocoa butter is where most of the fat is, it is best (for your health, at least!) to consume chocolate concoctions made from unsweetened natural cocoa powder. Make sure the cocoa powder has not been produced using the Dutch processing method. Avoid eating any chocolate processed with flavonoid-robbing alkali—if a quick inspection of the ingredients list on the back label reveals the word *alkali*, place the product back on the shelf.

THE SWEET BLOOD-PRESSURE-LOWERING SCIENCE OF DARK CHOCOLATE

How do we know that consuming flavanol-rich cocoa products (such as dark chocolate and cocoa beverages) has a measurable blood-pressure-lowering effect? From two types of research: large-scale observational studies of thousands of people that suggest an association between eating chocolate and lower blood pressure, as well as a number of randomized clinical trials proving that in fact eating dark chocolate causes a reduction in blood pressure. Let's take a peek at one of these observational studies to see just why scientists surmised that dark chocolate might have a medicinal effect (just as their ancient medical counterparts did).

Observational Research on Chocolate

A large German study showed that a little chocolate every day can cut your risk of a heart attack or stroke by a phenomenal 39 percent. Scientists at the German Institute for Human Nutrition in Nuthetal, Germany, followed the diet and health habits of nearly twenty thousand middle-aged Germans for ten years. Statistical analyses revealed that the people who ate about one square of chocolate every day had a significantly lower blood pressure compared to those indulging in the least amount of chocolate.[8] And a recent systematic meta-analysis combining data from seven large-scale observational studies (involving more than a hundred thousand subjects) came to a similar conclusion: the highest level of daily

NEW SWEDISH STUDY: CHOCOLATE CUTS STROKE RISK

A recent large-scale study out of Stockholm, Sweden, published in the journal *Neurology,* analyzed the association between chocolate consumption and risk of stroke by following almost forty thousand men for a period of ten years. It was found that men who consumed the most amount of chocolate (averaging about 63 grams of chocolate per week, which equates to about two Hershey's Kisses per day) had the lowest risk. Compared to the men who ate the least amount of chocolate, the chocolate eaters cut their risk of having a stroke by a whopping 17 percent! Now that's sweet.

Source: Larsson SC, Virtamo J, Wolk A. Chocolate consumption and risk of stroke: a prospective cohort of men and meta-analysis. *Neurology* 2012;79:1223–1229.

chocolate consumption was associated with a 37 percent reduction in risk of heart disease and a 29 percent decrease in risk of having a stroke compared to the lowest levels of chocolate consumption.[9]

Clinical Trial Data Show Cocoa's Potential Benefits

Once scientists suspect an association between an intervention (i.e., eating dark chocolate) and an outcome (in this case, lower blood pressure and better heart health), they need to go back to the lab and prove cause and effect. As you know by now, this is done using the gold standard of research techniques, the randomized, controlled clinical trial. The results of numerous such trials have revealed the sweet blood-pressure-lowering effect of a few daily bites of dark chocolate. For example, in a controlled Italian study of fifteen healthy adults, subjects ate either 100 grams (about 3.5 ounces) of dark chocolate or an equivalent amount of white chocolate daily for a two-week period. At the end of the trial, the dark-chocolate-eating group lowered their systolic pressure by an astounding 6 mm and diastolic by an equally impressive 4 mm Hg, compared to no change in those eating white chocolate.[10] Another randomized clinical trial of similar design comes from the same lab, but this time studied twenty people with high blood pressure who ate either 100 grams a day of flavanol-rich dark chocolate or the same amount of flavanol-free white chocolate. After two weeks, once again, those eating dark chocolate exhibited a phenomenal drop in systolic blood pressure of 12 mm Hg and 9 mm Hg diastolic compared to no blood pressure change in those eating white chocolate.[11]

A more recent study, published in the acclaimed *Journal of the American Medical Association*, supports the blood-pressure-lowering magic of dark chocolate. Researchers tested the effects on blood pressure of eating a small daily dose of dark chocolate, using forty-four men and women with prehypertension or stage 1 high blood pressure (not taking medication), over a period of eighteen weeks.[12] Subjects were divided into 2 groups. One group consumed a 30-calorie, 6.3 g piece of high-flavonoid dark chocolate (to give you an idea of how little that is, one Hershey's Kiss = 4.5 g) and the other a calorie-matched 5.6 g dose of polyphenol-free white chocolate daily. At the end of the study period, the patients who ate the dark chocolate exhibited a noteworthy reduction of systolic and diastolic pressures of 2.9/1.9 mm Hg—and this was without any accompanying drop in body weight. In contrast, those who ate the white chocolate had no change in blood pressure from baseline values.

Multiple Meta-analyses Support Big Benefits of Chocolate

Myriad meta-analyses of randomized experimental trials in humans continue to support the miraculous blood-pressure-lowering capabilities of dark chocolate. For example, a recent systematic review and meta-analysis of ten randomized clinical trials, comprising 297 participants, showed that systolic and diastolic blood pressure was lowered by 4.5/2.5 mm Hg, respectively, following daily cocoa ingestion (of varying amounts) for periods of two to eighteen weeks.[13] In 2007, a smaller meta-analysis, encompassing five randomized clinical trials and 173 subjects with normal blood pressure, revealed that flavanol-rich dark chocolate and cocoa lowered blood pressure numbers by an average of 4.7 mm Hg (systolic) and 2.8 mm Hg (diastolic).[14] Most recently, a meta-analysis of twenty clinical trials involving nearly nine hundred participants revealed a small but significant blood-pressure-lowering effect of daily dark cocoa intake (2.8 mm Hg systolic and 2.2 mm Hg diastolic).[15]

In Mice and Men: Rodent Studies Confirm Potential Benefits

New research in animals even supports the potential for cocoa to reduce blood pressure in hypertensive rats. When scientists randomly divided twenty male rats into two groups, one receiving tap water (control) and the other a solution of water with added cocoa extract, after seventeen weeks the cocoa-fed group reduced their systolic blood pressure by 10–15 mm Hg.[16] Another rodent study found that feeding hypertensive rats a large dose of high-polyphenol cocoa powder lowered their systolic blood pressure just as much as a medically effective dose of captopril, a common antihypertensive medication.[17] The science from both animal and human studies is clear: ingesting flavonoids in the form of dark chocolate is an effective lifestyle strategy for treating high blood pressure.

How Does Dark Chocolate Lower Blood Pressure?

Chocolate as blood pressure medicine? Sounds too good to be true! Here is the scientific explanation for how filling your daily chocolate prescription will soothe the savage arterial beast.

Method of attack #1: Chocolate is a natural ACE inhibitor. Recall from Chapter Two that the main blood-pressure-raising enzyme in your bloodstream is called angiotensin-converting enzyme (ACE). This enzyme is a prime target for blood-pressure-lowering prescription medications known as ACE inhibitors (such as quinapril), which work to lower pressure by stopping the enzyme's ability to convert the inert protein angiotensin I into the powerful arterial constrictor angiotensin II. In a recent randomized controlled trial, Swedish researchers discovered that chocolate has the same ACE-inhibiting effect as the prescription medication! In sixteen men and women who ate a daily dose of 75 grams (2.6 ounces) of dark chocolate containing 72 percent cocoa solids, ACE activity dropped an astonishing 18 percent in two weeks—a reduction similar to those observed with antihypertensive prescription medications.[18]

Method of attack #2: As you have learned, cocoa is a rich source of the main subclass of polyphenol flavonoids called flavan-3-ols. Flavan-3-ols have been shown to widen the arteries by increasing endothelial production of nitric oxide, the arterial relaxation chemical. Not only can cocoa components induce nitric oxide production directly, they can also improve the body's ability to manufacture it, as well as increase the body's ability to absorb it where it counts—deep down inside the arterial wall.[19]

Method of attack #3: As you know, dysfunction of the endothelium is a hallmark of people with high blood pressure. A little cocoa on a daily basis actually reverses endothelial dysfunction and enhances blood flow. (To prove this, scientists use a method called flow-mediated dilation. Numerous studies have shown enhanced blood flow following chocolate consumption using this technique.)[20,21,22]

Method of attack #4: Most people with high blood pressure have some degree of inflammation—chronic irritation that induces and perpetuates cardiovascular disease. Cocoa has been shown to quell the flames of inflammation, as evidenced by a reduction in a blood marker of inflammation called C-reactive protein (CRP). A study of more than two thousand healthy Italian subjects found that those eating dark chocolate showed a significantly lower CRP level than those who didn't eat chocolate.[23]

Method of attack #5: A heart attack or stroke is usually the result of a blood clot, which forms around ruptured plaque and blocks blood flow. Cells downstream of the clot die, and if enough heart muscle or brain cells die, the heart attack or stroke can be fatal. Chocolate thins the blood and makes the platelets less likely to stick together. This is because flavan-3-ols boost the production of nitric oxide, a potent platelet inhibitor.[24]

CHOCOLATE CAUTION

Chocolate is an energy-dense food, meaning it contains a lot of calories in just a few bites. Chocolate bars are made from cocoa solids (the fat-free, low-calorie portion where the health benefits lie), as well as plenty of cocoa fat and added sugar. The fat in cocoa is saturated, so it can raise the level of "bad" (LDL) cholesterol. (Albeit, over half of the saturated fat in cocoa butter is stearic acid, which is cholesterol neutral.) And fat isn't the only health culprit lurking in most chocolate—sugar is also a dietary evil, one that the AHA recently added to its "blacklist"—joining the ranks of saturated fat, trans fat, dietary cholesterol, and sodium—of foods to limit for better heart health.)

Added sugars are used by food companies to sweeten convenience foods such as soda, candy, fruit drinks, dairy products (including sweetened yogurts, sweetened milk, and ice cream), cereals, and desserts. The average American takes in about 22 teaspoons of added sugar daily. This translates into a daily addition of 355 empty calories. According to the AHA, extra sugar intake can contribute to the development of high blood pressure, high triglycerides, obesity, insulin resistance, and type 2 diabetes. The AHA recommends a daily maximum of 100 calories from added sugar for women (25 grams, or 6 teaspoons) and 150 calories for men (37 grams, or 9 teaspoons).

So just how much added sugar is in two squares of dark chocolate? There are approximately 13 grams of sugar (3 teaspoons) in a 1-ounce portion of a typical dark chocolate bar. So don't worry—your chocolate indulgence is well below the recommended daily intake.

One way around the sugar problem is to consume unsweetened natural cocoa powder—a polyphenol-packed, low-calorie, fat-free version of the chocolate bar. Add your own sweetener and low-fat dairy or soy milk, and you have a delicious diet food with all the blood-pressure-lowering benefits of dark chocolate without the "bad" fat and excess calories.

The takeaway message is that this blood pressure medicine needs to be savored in small amounts. Eating too much dark chocolate can add pounds on the scale, which would negate the blood pressure benefits.

FILLING THE PRESCRIPTION

Let's learn a lesson from the indigenous Kuna Islanders and tap into the ultimate health food—dark, deliciously satisfying chocolate, the "food of the gods." Each day, aim for 2 tablespoons of natural unsweetened cocoa powder (not Dutch-processed), or 1 to 2 ounces of dark chocolate.

Remember, to satisfy your chocolate craving and lower your pressure simultaneously, think real cocoa. Natural unsweetened cocoa powder has the highest concentration of flavan-3-ols compared to other chocolate products (followed by unsweetened baking chocolate), plus is low in sugar, fat, and calories, so favor this chocolate choice over chocolate bars when possible. And don't forget that milk chocolate and chocolate syrup rank lowest on the antioxidant scale, so avoid choosing them for your chocolate splurge.[25]

Another bonus of eating cocoa powder is the fact that it adds to your daily potassium intake as well—3 tablespoons provide approximately 80 mg of potassium.

Type	Amount	Calories
Unsweetened natural cocoa powder	2 tablespoons	24
Unsweetened baking chocolate squares	1 square (1 oz square)	140
Dark chocolate bars (at least 70 percent cocoa):	2 squares	115
Lindt Extra Dark Chocolate (85 percent cacao)	2 squares	115
Trader Joe's Dark Chocolate (72 percent cacao)	½ a bar (6 squares or approximately 24 grams)	140

Here are six tips for adding dark chocolate to your day:

1. Try a nightly cup of steaming, decadent homemade hot chocolate. Put 2 heaping spoonfuls of natural unsweetened cocoa powder into a mug, along with a touch of sweetener (you might consider a sugar substitute), add soy milk, mix, and microwave. Top with fat-free whipped topping and you have a delicious, chocolaty, super-heart-healthy and blood-pressure-lowering sweet treat.

2. Look for single-origin dark chocolate products. Madagascar and Java cacao beans have been shown to contain double the flavan-3-ols compared to beans from other areas. (You should also know that, sad to say, child labor is a common practice in the cocoa plantations of Africa. Both Mars and Ferrero have pledged to use 100 percent certified sustainable cocoa for their products—a standard that less than 35 percent of the world's cocoa supply meets. Although certification is no guarantee the cocoa was harvested without child labor, it is a step in the right direction.)[26]

3. Bake with unsweetened cocoa powder or unsweetened baking chocolate squares (both top the antioxidant scale).

4. Melt a few semisweet chocolate chips, pour the chocolate over a banana, and top with a dollop of fat-free whipped cream.

5. Savor one or two pieces of a dark chocolate bar (at least 70 percent cacao) with a nightly cup of tea.

6. Buy a bag of pre-portioned dark chocolate squares and indulge in a daily treat without affecting your waistline. Take them with you on trips and to restaurants so you can enjoy your chocolate blood pressure medicine on the go!

Chocolate has been consumed and enjoyed by humans for millennia. Isn't it sweet to know that this food will help your blood pressure go down?

You have learned how formidable the plant chemicals are that lie buried within this superfood, and how they help your cardiovascular health. The Blood Pressure Down plan is not about deprivation but instead urges you to tap into Mother Nature's spectacular bounty of natural blood-pressure-lowering foods—in just the right dosage—to help you both extend and enjoy your life. So relish your daily dose of strong, divinely delicious chocolate—perhaps in combination with a soothing cup of green tea or a glass of your favorite red wine—and take delight in your blood pressure medicine, enjoying life and lowering your millimeters of mercury the Blood Pressure Down way.

Step 8: Drink Red Wine

R̶x̶ Drink a Glass of Red Wine with Dinner

Why is it that the region of the United States consuming the least amount of alcohol—much of the southern United States extending west into Texas and Oklahoma—is known as "Stroke Alley"? Could it be that a little alcohol, more specifically a daily tipple of red wine, protects against heart and circulatory disease? Perhaps. In this chapter, I'll explain how drinking alcohol in small amounts with a meal can lower blood pressure. But first you need to be aware that of all the steps in the Blood Pressure Down plan, this one is the most precarious.

Alcohol is a tricky medication. Its physiological, metabolic, and psychological effects are complex. Both excessive alcohol intake and alcohol abstinence—the opposite ends of the alcohol consumption spectrum—have been proven to raise blood pressure.[1] So we are going to aim for that sweet spot in the middle. A moderate amount of alcohol is healthful, but anything more than two drinks a day (or what's called "episodic binge drinking," defined as five or more drinks for men, four or more for women, in a two-hour time frame) is toxic to the heart and arteries, contributes to high blood pressure, and shortens the life span.[2] In the words of Henry Fielding, the eighteenth-century British playwright and novelist, "Wine is a turncoat; first a friend and then an enemy." The good news is that you can reverse the blood-pressure-raising effect of high amounts of alcohol simply by moderating intake. So proceed with caution in following this step, and fill the prescription only if you and your personal physician know that you can drink responsibly.

WINE: THE GIFT OF THE GODS

Wine has soaked through the pages of history for millennia, praised for its medicinal, social, and nutritional value. The medicinal use of wine dates back as far as 2200 B.C., making it the oldest known medicine. The ancient Greeks praised wine as a gift of the gods: Homer's love for grapes and wine permeates his poetry, and the early physician Hippocrates used wine as part of almost all his recorded therapeutic cures. Fast-forward to the present day, and the scientific evidence is crystal clear: individuals who consume a small amount of red wine daily with meals experience a 20 to 30 percent reduction in risk of death from heart disease and stroke compared to both teetotalers and those who drink alcohol in excess.[3]

ALCOHOL: THE CASE FOR MODERATE CONSUMPTION

So just how cardioprotective is sensible drinking? A strong body of scientific evidence suggests that light to moderate alcohol

ALCOHOL AND BLOOD PRESSURE: A DOUBLE-EDGED SWORD

The general medical consensus is that drinking a small amount of red wine daily with food is part of the lifestyle prescription for preventing the onset of high blood pressure. If you already have high blood pressure and currently drink more than moderate amounts of alcohol on a daily basis, then you should know that your alcohol consumption is a contributing factor to your disease. Cutting back on your daily intake and switching over to red wine will lower your pressure.

consumption reduces risk of death from a heart attack by a phenomenal 30 to 50 percent for both men and women.[4] Considering that heart attacks and stroke are the leading causes of death in this country and that those of us with high pressure are at greatest risk, it would behoove all of us to raise a glass to heart health.

Drinking for heart health also means drinking in moderation. The World Health Organization estimates that 16 percent of global high blood pressure cases occur due to excessive alcohol intake. Above approximately 15 grams a day (around the amount of alcohol in 5 ounces of wine), each 10 grams of alcohol consumed is associated with a 1 mm Hg rise in blood pressure. The great news is that this aberration is largely reversible with a few weeks of abstinence or reduction in alcohol intake.

RED FLAG WARNINGS

- Alcohol can interact with prescription medications.
- For women at risk of breast cancer, any amount of alcohol increases risk.
- For pregnant women, there is no safe level of alcohol consumption.
- Avoid alcohol if you have been diagnosed with cardiomyopathy or cardiac arrhythmias.
- Avoid alcohol if you have a personal or family history of substance abuse.

How Much Alcohol Does It Take to Raise Blood Pressure?

When it comes to alcohol use and blood pressure, it's about both quantity and pattern. There is clearly a connection between the amount of alcohol consumed and high blood pressure. We have known this since 1915, when researchers found that wine-drinking French troops serving on the Western Front in World War I had higher-than-normal blood pressure readings compared to other nationalities fighting.

Frequency of consumption also plays a role. Episodic binge drinking raises blood pressure, whereas the same amount of alcohol spread out over the course of a week in moderate daily servings and taken with food lowers pressure. The *type* of alcohol, though, does not seem to make a difference when it comes to raising blood pressure. Researchers in Australia studied whether high daily amounts of alcohol, in the form of red wine or beer, affected blood pressure in twenty-four healthy young men who were assigned to four weeks of drinking approximately 40 grams of alcohol per day (almost 4 glasses of wine or beer). Both the red wine and the beer resulted in an increase of systolic blood pressure, by 3 mm Hg in the wine drinkers and 2 mm Hg in the beer drinkers.[5] The takeaway: drinking too much of any kind of alcohol—even heart-healthy red wine—can cause your pressure to rise.

WHAT IS A "DRINK"?

The USDA dietary guidelines define one drink as 12 ounces of beer, 5 ounces of wine, 1½ ounces of 80-proof spirits, or 1 ounce of 100-proof spirits—all of which contain approximately 12 to 15 grams of alcohol. Moderate alcohol consumption is defined as one drink per day for women and up to two drinks per day for men. Heavy drinking is anything that exceeds this amount.

The relationship between alcohol and high blood pressure can be visually represented as a J-shaped curve: heavy drinkers exhibit the greatest risk, light to moderate drinkers exhibit the lowest risk, and abstainers have an intermediate risk.[6] The relationship between heavy drinking and an increase in blood pressure follows what scientists call a "direct, dose-response" pattern—meaning that the more you drink, the greater your risk, particularly when alcohol intake exceeds two drinks per day.[7,8,9]

Large-Scale Studies Prove Too Much Alcohol Is Bad for Blood Pressure

We learned decades ago from the Nurses' Health Study that a daily alcohol consumption over 20 grams per day (that's about 1½ glasses of wine) increases women's risk of high blood pressure, with the risk progressively increasing with intake. Drinking 20 to 34 grams of alcohol (about two or three drinks) per day increased risk of high blood pressure by an astronomical 40 percent, while drinking more than three drinks (more than 35 grams of alcohol) a day increased risk by 90 percent.[10]

The Atherosclerosis Risk in Communities Study, which observed health and dietary patterns in more than eight thousand healthy, middle-aged men and women for a period of six years, confirmed that alcohol consumption of more than two drinks per day is associated with great risk for high blood pressure.[11,12] It also revealed that drinking outside of mealtimes increased blood pressure risk more than drinking with food.

Moderate Drinking Cuts Heart Attacks

If you have been diagnosed with high blood pressure, you can still drink—a little. You should know that data from more than fourteen thousand male doctors drawn from the Physicians' Health Study support the heart health benefits of light to moderate drinking in men with previously diagnosed high blood pressure. Over a five-and-a-half-year study period, moderate drinkers with high blood pressure had a 44 percent reduced risk of dying from a heart attack compared to the doctors with high blood pressure who rarely or never drank.[13] But don't overdose on your liquid medicine; as you have learned, excessive alcohol intake clearly raises blood pressure, so make sure not to exceed the recommended daily limit of one to two drinks per day.[14]

DRINKING TOO MUCH? CUTTING BACK CAN CUT PRESSURE

Clearly, drinking excessively is a major cause of high blood pressure. So what happens if you are a hypertensive drinker and you cut back on your alcohol intake? Your pressure drops, according to a meta-analysis of fifteen randomized clinical trials designed to answer just this question. The analysis involved more than twenty-two hundred heavy drinkers (defined as consuming three to six alcoholic drinks per day). Lowering alcohol intake to moderate levels resulted in an average drop in systolic pressure of 3.31 mm Hg and a drop in diastolic pressure of 2.04 mm Hg. The takeaway message? Elevation in blood pressure as a result of excess alcohol intake is largely reversible with two to four weeks of abstinence or significant moderation. The scientific consensus appears to be that reducing excessive alcohol intake can lower blood pressure as much as 4 mm Hg on average.

Sources: Xin X, He J, Frontini MG, et al. Effects of alcohol reduction on blood pressure: a meta-analysis of randomized controlled trials. *Hypertens* 2001;38:1112–1117; Kodavali L, Townsend RR. Alcohol and its relationship to blood pressure. *Curr Hypertens Rep.* 2006;8(4):338–344.

Cheers to a Long and Healthy Life

Without question, the scientific data are clear: regular, light to moderate drinking with meals guards against heart and vascular disease and lengthens life. Remember the Nurses' Health Study, in which women who practiced all six low-risk behaviors cut their risk of developing high blood pressure by a whopping 78 percent?[15] One of the six sensational lifestyle factors was alcohol intake of up to 10 grams per day (about one glass of wine).

CURB HIGH BLOOD PRESSURE WITH A DAILY TOAST OF RED WINE

So what kind of alcohol should you choose? You have probably heard red wine touted as a liquid blood pressure medicine. Indeed, red wine is best for disease prevention, as moderate wine drinkers have the lowest risk of death from all causes.[16] Let's take a closer look at the heart-healthy benefits of red wine.

Scientists in Greece analyzed the lifelong drinking habits of nearly six hundred elderly men and women from the Mediterranean islands and discovered that those people who drank an average of one to two glasses of red wine per day were 13 percent less likely to have high blood pressure than their teetotaler comrades.[17] Although all types of alcoholic drinks, taken daily and in small amounts, are associated with a lower risk of heart disease, red wine offers the greatest cardioprotection.[18] This is why the Blood Pressure Down plan includes a small amount of red wine as your alcoholic beverage prescription. Next up, we'll see why.

> When it comes to wine, the American Heart Association is very clear on the ideal amount for blood pressure regulation: no more than one glass (5 ounces) a day for women and no more than two glasses for men.

What's in Red Wine That Lowers Pressure?

Red wine contains two substances thought to contribute to its blood-pressure-lowering power: ethanol (alcohol) and an array of powerful antioxidants called polyphenols (including resveratrol and the procyanidins). Numerous studies have established that ethanol helps combat circulatory disease by causing the arteries to relax and widen, allowing more blood to flow through and blood pressure to drop.

In addition to its vasodilatory effect, ethanol also acts as a solvent for the polyphenols, increasing the amount of these important nutrients that are extracted during the processing of the wine and making them readily available for your intestine to absorb.[19]

Powering Down Pressure with Polyphenols

Polyphenols, the alcohol-free portion of red wine, are the crucial chemicals that set red wine above and beyond other types of alcohol in terms of the benefits for your heart and arteries. So let's take a closer look at how these plant chemicals affect your pressure (Figure 11.1). Polyphenols are antioxidants, natural plant substances that ward off disease. The polyphenols contained in red wine can be divided into two main groups: *flavonoids* (flavan-3-ols—which you may remember from our dark chocolate lesson—flavonols, and anthocyanins) and *nonflavonoids* (stilbenes, or resveratrol, and phenolic acids (Figure 11.1).[20] There are more than five hundred different types of antioxidants found in grapes, most of which are located in the skin and seeds.[21] (Note that flavonoids are located in both the skin and the seeds of grapes, whereas resveratrol, the most famous nonflavonoid, is found only in the skin.)

To tap into wine's huge cache of powerful polyphenols, be sure to pick red over white. Red wine has ten times the polyphenol content of white wine, because it is fermented with the macerated skins and seeds of the grape. (White wine is made by quickly pressing the juice away from the grape solids.) On average, red wine contains between six and nine times the amount of polyphenols that white wine does.

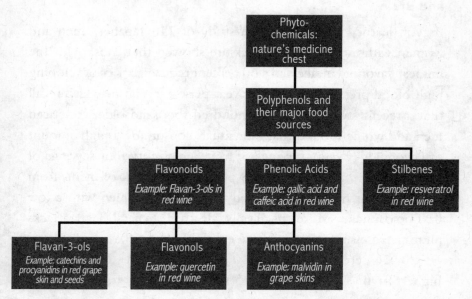

Figure 11.1   Red wine contains primarily the nonflavonoid polyphenols (stilbenes and phenolic acids) and the polyphenol flavonoids (flavan-3-ols, flavonols, and anthocyanins).

Now, not all red wines are created equal; they vary both in the type of polyphenols they contain and in the polyphenol concentration. So which red wines have the highest polyphenol content? This depends on many factors. The antioxidant content can vary considerably among different grapes from different regions, and even within wines made from the same type of grape. In general, wines made with grape solids during the maceration process, as well as those made from grapes exposed to greater environmental stress, have higher polyphenol content. Grapevines grown in higher-elevation vineyards and those exposed to fungal infection produce grapes with greater levels of resveratrol (the nonflavonoid type of polyphenol), because plants produce resveratrol in response to stresses such as infection and cold and wet environments. By contrast, grapevines that face stresses such as harsh sun exposure and nutrient deprivation produce grapes with more flavonoids.

Greater Flavonoids, Lower Pressure, Healthier Heart and Brain

As you learned in Chapter 9, a study of 745 Japanese men and women without high blood pressure showed that those with the highest flavonoid intake had a 60 percent reduced risk of developing high blood pressure over a four-year period.[22] You may also recall that a recent study of nearly a hundred thousand older American men and women found that individuals consuming a high amount of flavonoids (twenty servings of fruit and twenty-four servings of vegetables per week) had an 18 percent lower risk of dying from cardiovascular troubles compared to men and women with a low flavonoid intake. More specifically, death from fatal heart attacks plummeted even further in those eating the most flavonoids, dropping by 25 percent (men) and 40 percent (women). Men with the highest flavonoid intake were 37 percent less likely to experience a fatal stroke.[23]

Tap into the Power of Procyanidins:
Red Wine's Superflavonoids

While resveratrol has received the most attention, it actually is the procyanidin flavonoids (condensed tannins) in red wine that have proven to be the most potent polyphenol for our blood vessels. Scientists suspect that of all the polyphenols, the procyanidins have the most positive effect on the inner lining of the arterial wall, the endothelium. Grape seeds are the primary source of procyanidins, and the procyanidin content of red wines varies with the method of winemaking and the type of grape used.[24] For the red wines with the highest procyanidin content, look for those from Sardinia (in Italy) and southwestern France (which, interestingly, is the area with the greatest longevity among the French population).

RESVERATROL AND PROCYANIDIN:
WHICH RED WINES HAVE THE MOST?

The red wine varieties with the most resveratrol include pinot noir, malbec, and petite sirah. For highest procyanidin content, it's best to drink the deeply colored reds—in general, cabernet sauvignon is your best bet.

Resveratrol, a Fountain of Youth?

Resveratrol has been on the public's radar lately because of research linking large doses of resveratrol to an increased life span in mice. Harvard scientists have shown that feeding resveratrol to mice can stimulate the synthesis of proteins called sirtuins that slow aging. Sounds great, right? Well, yes and no. The problem is in the translation. A human would have to drink a hundred to a thousand bottles of red wine per day to receive a resveratrol dosage equal to what was administered to the mice—not exactly a realistic anti-aging plan!

Blood pressure, however, is a different story. Studies of humans have shown that the amount of resveratrol in a single daily glass of red wine is enough to stimulate the production of the blood-pressure-lowering superchemical nitric oxide.[25]

The Blood-Pressure-Lowering Power of the Purple Majesty

The blood vessel benefits of a daily tipple of red wine are well documented and are attributed to several actions involving both the alcohol and the antioxidant components. Here is a synopsis of just how drinking red wine in moderation can benefit your arteries.

Method of attack #1: The resveratrol, procyanidins, and quercetin in red wine stimulate the production of the vasodilator nitric oxide. As you remember, nitric oxide relaxes blood vessels, reduces blood pressure, and improves vascular health. (Recall that nitric oxide is in short supply in blood pressure patients—a major contributing factor to constricted and diseased vessels.)[26] Regular moderate wine consumption also increases the sensitivity of the smooth muscle cells to the relaxation effect of nitric oxide.[27]

What kind of red wine is best for enhancing vasodilation? An Italian study found that red wine produced in small oak barrels and large wood barrels has statistically greater vasodilatory effects (in both people with normal blood pressure and high blood pressure) than wine produced in large steel tanks.[28] The authors concluded that red wines produced in wooden barrels (a technique widely used in France and Italy) contain greater amounts of quercetin and tannic acid, which translates into greater blood pressure benefits.

Method of attack #2: Drinking a little bit of alcohol in moderation can also help you regulate your blood sugar level and lower your risk of developing type 2 diabetes—which, as you've learned, is important for controlling your blood pressure. A meta-analysis of fifteen large-scale studies, involving nearly 370,000 individuals, revealed that moderate drinkers cut their risk of developing type 2 diabetes by 30 percent when compared to abstainers. (In this case,

---

A DAILY GLASS OF WINE CUTS STROKE RISK IN WOMEN

Considering that the majority of strokes are caused by high blood pressure, you may want to consider raising a toast to your brain health. Recent research published in the journal *Stroke* has shown that 5 to 15 grams of alcohol (the amount in ½ to 1½ glasses of wine) cuts risk of stroke in women by 17 to 21 percent. A significantly greater risk of stroke was shown in women consuming alcohol in excess of 36 grams per day (the amount in approximately three glasses of wine), however, highlighting the fact that the difference between drinking in moderation and drinking in excess is the difference between preventing disease and causing disease.

Source: Jiminez M, Chiuve SE, Glynn RJ, et al. Alcohol consumption and risk of stroke in women. *Stroke* 2012;43. DOI:10.1161/STROKEAHA.111.639435/-/DC1.

"moderate" was defined as anywhere between 6 and 48 grams of alcohol a day, or between ½ and 3½ glasses of wine.)[29]

One reason moderate alcohol consumption can have a favorable effect on your blood sugar is because drinking lightly increases your cells' sensitivity to insulin. When your cells become more sensitive to insulin, your body metabolizes sugar better, at least for twelve to twenty-four hours following alcohol ingestion. This greater insulin sensitivity helps to thwart metabolic syndrome, the constellation of metabolic disorders that accelerates atherosclerosis and is often a precursor to type 2 diabetes. A one-drink-a-day habit has been shown to lessen the likelihood of developing metabolic syndrome by a phenomenal 40 percent.[30]

Method of attack #3: As you know, most people with high blood pressure have some degree of inflammation in their arterial wall. Regular wine consumption has been shown to soothe that inflammation by inducing the release of anti-inflammatory chemicals into the arteries. In a randomized clinical trial of sixty-seven

Spanish men, subjects received either a daily dose of 30 grams of alcohol in the form of regular red wine (containing both alcohol and polyphenols), dealcoholized red wine (red wine polyphenols alone), or 30 grams of alcohol in the form of gin (only alcohol) for four weeks. Results showed that the regular red wine—the combination of ethanol and polyphenols—was superior in its anti-inflammatory effects compared to the other singular components.[31]

Method of attack #4: Red wine may help you win the battle of the bulge. As the *Journal of Biological Chemistry* notes, Korean scientists recently discovered a compound in red wine called piceatannol (it's a metabolite of resveratrol) that actually blocks the ability of immature fat cells to grow.[32] So red wine and this cousin of resveratrol could potentially help you to lose those five pounds and cut your blood pressure down to size.

RED WINE CAUTION

I cannot emphasize this enough: if your pressure is high and you drink in excess, your drinking is *raising* your millimeters of mercury. Overdrinking can severely damage your health and put you at risk of stroke, heart disease, certain forms of cancer, and liver cirrhosis, as well as alcohol abuse and alcoholism. Excessive drinking can also shorten life span. If you drink in excess, cut back on the alcohol and you will lower your blood pressure, prevent these dire consequences, and extend your life.

If you are not capable of drinking in moderation, then abstinence is clearly the best blood pressure medicine for you. When it comes to red wine consumption, the difference between drinking in moderation and drinking in excess is the difference between lowering your pressure and increasing it. *Only include the red wine prescription in your Blood Pressure Down plan if you and your personal physician mutually agree that you can drink safely and hit that sweet spot of one or two drinks per day.*

FILLING THE PRESCRIPTION

In this chapter, you have learned about the benefits and dangers of drinking wine for blood pressure regulation. If you are able to drink responsibly, you should feel free to enjoy a daily glass or two of red wine with food as part of a heart-healthy lifestyle. I urge you to take the time to sit down to a relaxing dinner of deliciously fresh whole food, artfully prepared and accompanied by your favorite glass of vino. In addition to helping you savor your food, red wine—a veritable cauldron of plant chemicals—can lower your blood pressure, not to mention calm your nerves, raise your "good" (HDL) cholesterol, increase your insulin sensitivity, and lower arterial inflammation.

Your wine blood pressure medication is most effective when taken daily and in moderation (just like your exercise prescription), and preferably with food. So take the time out of your hectic day to savor your family, your friends, your fresh and beautiful meal, and a toast to a long and healthy low-pressure life!

Step 9: Take Four Supplements

 Take Vitamin D₃, CoQ10, Fish Oil, and a Cup of Low-Sodium Vegetable Juice Every Day

By now you know that healthful lifestyle changes such as losing weight and following a low-sodium diet rich in potassium, calcium, and magnesium form the foundation of the Blood Pressure Down plan. While nutritional supplements should not be the first-line treatment for high blood pressure, there is an emerging body of scientific support for the safety and efficacy of a select few supplements in lowering blood pressure. You should know, however, that this step in the Blood Pressure Down plan is most likely the weakest link in the chain, as there is still controversy regarding the efficacy of supplements. That said, read on to decide for yourself how they may or may not fit into your blood-pressure-lowering strategy.

THE CASE FOR SUPPLEMENTATION

The fact is that few people eat perfectly. As an adjunct to a healthy lifestyle, supplements can compensate for our dietary imperfections by filling in the gaps on those days when we can't get enough of the blood-pressure-friendly nutrients we need. As a nutritionist, I always advise my patients to obtain their nutrient requirements from food rather than pills, but there are a few times when a supplement truly comes in handy. The following four supplements have made the cut—there is enough scientific evidence (albeit some of it questionable) to merit a spot on the Blood Pressure Down daily checklist.

1. Vitamin D_3 (1,000 to 2,000 IU/day—only if your doctor has deemed your blood level to be deficient)
2. Coenzyme Q10 (100 to 300 mg/day)
3. Omega-3 fish oil (1–2 grams of high-quality fish oil per day—with your doctor's consent)
4. Low-sodium vegetable juice (1 cup/day)

Let's examine each supplement in greater depth and learn just how popping these pills and downing your vegetable shot can help in your quest to get—and keep—your blood pressure down.

TO D OR NOT TO D . . . THAT IS THE QUESTION

Vitamin D is an unusual nutrient because it is a vitamin but acts more like a hormone. The term "vitamin D" refers to two types of inactive provitamins, known as the D precursors: D_2 (ergocalciferol) and D_3 (cholecalciferol), which are converted to their active form by the liver and kidneys. We obtain vitamin D from food, but we also manufacture it when our skin cells are exposed to the sun (that's why vitamin D is sometimes called the "sunshine vitamin"). The only naturally rich food sources of vitamin D are fatty fish such as salmon, tuna, and sardines. Vitamin D is also found in fortified dairy products, some soy products, fortified ready-to-eat cereals, and certain brands of fortified orange juice. (If you haven't guessed already, "fortified" means that the vitamin D was added in artificially.)

So what does vitamin D have to do with blood pressure? First, people with diagnosed hypertension are much more likely to have a low level of vitamin D than people with normal blood pressure.[1] And a comprehensive meta-analysis of randomized clinical trials involving more than four hundred subjects has shown that taking vitamin D supplements causes a decline in systolic blood pressure of approximately 2.4 mm Hg.[2] Why? Let's take a look at the physiological role of vitamin D and its metabolic partner, calcium, as well as D's complex relationship with the renin system.

Method of attack #1: As you learned in Chapter Eight, vitamin D and calcium go together like peanut butter and jelly. Your digestive system needs both of them in the intestinal tract in order for your body to absorb calcium. Vitamin D is also necessary to regulate the amount of calcium circulating in the bloodstream. When it comes to blood pressure, calcium and vitamin D must be balanced to keep your vessels relaxed and flexible. In fact, a recent study out of the Czech Republic found that people with the lowest vitamin D level in their blood had the stiffest arteries.[3] The scientists surmised that without enough vitamin D to regulate calcium, excess calcium gets deposited in the inner wall of the arteries, stiffening and hardening them.

Method of attack #2: Recall from Chapter Two that renin is the hormone produced by the kidneys that leads to conversion of angiotensin I to angiotensin II—the most powerful vasoconstrictor there is. Vitamin D suppresses the kidney's synthesis of renin[4] and acts like a natural ACE inhibitor by putting the brakes on the entire renin-angiotensin system, thereby lowering the amount of the volatile blood-pressure-raising angiotensin II.[5] Vitamin D in the bloodstream also helps to calm the smooth muscle cells in the arteries, keeping blood pressure down.[6]

How Low Is Too Low?

Have your doctor test your vitamin D level. Vitamin D measurements are reported in either nanograms per milliliter (ng/mL) or nanomoles per liter (nmol/L). The scientific consensus points to a blood level of vitamin D that is between 35 and 40 ng/mL (90 and 100 nmol/L) for optimal health. According to the National Institutes of Health, a value of less than 15 ng/mL (37.5 nmol/L) means you have a vitamin D deficiency. People with hypertension are more likely to have low vitamin D levels compared to healthy people.

Getting enough vitamin D from food and sunshine is ideal, but this is hard for many of us to accomplish. Why? Natural vitamin D is found in just a few foods (including wild salmon, swordfish, and cod liver oil), and for those of us who reside in northern climates, it is nearly impossible to get enough sun in the winter months. The good news is that if your levels of vitamin D are indeed low, taking a daily vitamin D_3 supplement will help—that's why I suggest you take 1,000–2,000 IU of vitamin D (under your doctor's supervision). And read the label to make sure that the supplement you are taking provides vitamin D_3 (the form of the vitamin called cholecalciferol) and not D_2 (ergocalciferol). Results from a new meta-analysis—hot off the presses—has confirmed that vitamin D_3 is more effective at increasing blood levels of the sunshine vitamin than the D_2 form of the supplement.[7]

CAPITALIZING ON COENZYME Q10

What is coenzyme Q10? Nicknamed CoQ10, this is a naturally occurring vitamin-like substance located within the cells' mitochondria, the power-producing part of the cell. CoQ10 is important both for energy metabolism and as a potent antioxidant. CoQ10 is also known as *ubiquinone*, because of its ubiquitous distribution in the human body—with its highest concentration in the heart.

We have known for decades that people with high blood pressure tend to have low cellular levels of CoQ10, suggesting that a lack of this enzyme may hinder blood pressure regulation.[8] So it makes sense that many doctors have wondered if supplementing with CoQ10 could in fact help lower blood pressure. Exciting new research is backing up this claim. In an Australian meta-analysis of twelve clinical trials involving 362 people with high blood pressure, CoQ10 supplements were shown to lower blood pressure significantly—by an average of 17 mm Hg systolic and 8 mm Hg diastolic—without any side effects.[9] You should know, however, that not all the research is so optimistic. A recent well-designed clinical trial failed to show any positive blood-pressure-lowering effect of 200 mg of CoQ10 per day (for twelve weeks) in hypertensive subjects.[10] Despite these findings, the fact is that CoQ10 is an extremely safe supplement. Hence, for the time being, I suggest using the supplement until this controversy is clarified and more definitive data on its efficacy for blood pressure reduction are available.

CoQ10: How Much Is Enough?

How much should you take to get any potential blood-pressure-lowering effect? The jury is still out on the exact dosage for the best results, since each person has a different response and different brands are absorbed differently. Another complicating factor is statin medication, prescription drugs used to lower "bad" (LDL) cholesterol. Statins work by inhibiting production of cholesterol in the liver. But they also inhibit CoQ10 production—LDL and CoQ10 share a common pathway for synthesis. If you are taking statin drugs, you may need a higher dosage of CoQ10 supplements. I suggest that you start with anywhere from 100 to 300 mg/day (under your doctor's supervision).

Method of attack: How does CoQ10 lower your blood pressure? One common cause of high blood pressure is a state called oxidative stress. This is a situation where excessive amounts of marauding, highly destructive molecules called free radicals attack the fragile endothelium, impairing the blood vessels' ability to relax and dilate. (Free radicals are formed through excessive exposure to radiation and pollution, and are also naturally produced through metabolic processes.)

What protection does your body have against destructive free radicals? The answer is antioxidants, otherwise known as free radical scavengers. You have probably heard of antioxidants as they relate to preventing cancer, but the truth is that they are important for your blood pressure too. The body uses antioxidants to stop free radicals before they start a chain reaction of oxidation that damages cells and DNA. CoQ10 is a potent chain-breaking antioxidant with the proven ability to counteract the constriction of the arteries by free radicals, thus fighting off oxidative stress and lowering blood pressure.[11]

FISHING FOR LOWER BLOOD PRESSURE

Now we're going to learn about the blood-pressure-lowering power of another nutritional superstar: essential fatty acids. Nutritionists often refer to these unsaturated fats as "protective." There are two main groups of fatty acids, both essential for life: omega-3 fatty acids and omega-6 fatty acids. The omega-3s are further broken down into two types: short-chain omega-3 fats (alpha-linolenic acid, or ALA), found in land-based plants, and long-chain omega-3s (eicosapentaenoic acid, or EPA, and docosahexaenoic acid, or DHA), found in marine life, both of which are known to enhance human health.

The names are complicated, but for the purposes of the Blood Pressure Down plan, all you need to know is that the omega-3 fatty acids confer extremely powerful heart and vascular protective effects. You need to make a concerted effort daily to eat more plant-derived short-chain omega-3 fat (ALA) and marine-derived long-chain omega-3s (EPA and DHA). What's the best way to pack your diet with these healthy fats? The richest sources of ALA are seed oils (such as canola oil), walnuts, flaxseed, and chia seeds.

As for the marine-derived omega-3s, our primary source is fish, especially the fatty types of fish that swim in the deep, cold waters of the sea. If you are a vegetarian or vegan, you might consider taking algae-derived DHA supplements.

Omega-3s: How Much Is Enough?

For overall good health, wellness professionals typically advocate at least 2 grams of ALA and 500 mg of EPA/DHA daily.[12] Along these same lines, the American Heart Association recommends that for heart health benefits, Americans should strive to eat at least two omega-3-rich fish meals per week (which equates to the 500 mg/day guideline). Unfortunately, most Americans eat far too little of this superfat, averaging less than 100 mg/day. On the Blood Pressure Down plan, the goal is to eat at least two fish meals each week.

The best sources of the omega-3 fatty acids EPA and DHA are the cold-water fatty fish, such as salmon, mackerel, lake trout, herring, sardines, and albacore tuna.

In addition to eating fish, research has shown that taking omega-3 fish oil in supplement form can lower your blood pressure. Before we dive into the science, let's look at exactly what essential fats are, and why we need to eat less of one type and more of another.

Your Health Is in the Balance

Although some essential fatty acids come from meat and fish, most come from plants (including water plants such as phytoplankton and algae). Linoleic acid (LA), or omega-6 fat, is found mainly in seeds, nuts, and legumes. While omega-6s are essential for your health, most Americans already get an oversupply from the omega-6-rich vegetable oils that pervade our food supply. Safflower oil and cottonseed oil, for example, are cheap oils widely used in the food service and snack food industries. Be on the lookout for cottonseed oil in packaged foods—it's often hiding in potato chips, peanut butter,

---

CUT STROKE RISK: EAT FISH

Omega-3 fats from fish are good for the heart, the blood vessels, and the brain. That's the news out of Sweden, where researchers examined the fish-eating habits of nearly thirty-five thousand women over a period of ten years. Women who consumed three or more fish meals a week cut their risk of stroke by 33 percent compared to their non-fish-eating counterparts. Note that in Sweden, some types of fish, such as herring, are typically salted. There was no association between eating salted fish and a reduced risk of stroke—reaffirming what we already know about the harmful attributes of sodium.

Source: Larsson SC, Virtamo J, Wolk A. Fish consumption and risk of stroke in Swedish women. *Am J Clin Nutr* 2011;93:487–493.

---

boxed cereals, cookies and crackers, breads, salad dressings, mayonnaise, and marinades. Cottonseed oil is often blended with other oils and may be listed as "vegetable oil," "vegetable oil shortening," or "hydrogenated vegetable oil" on food labels.

At the same time as we are eating too much omega-6 fat, we get an undersupply of healthful omega-3 fats, which are not nearly as plentiful in our food supply. This troublesome fatty acid imbalance—too many omega-6s and too few omega-3s—leads to negative health ramifications. One such problem is inflammation. The body uses essential fatty acids to produce hormone-like substances called eicosanoids, which regulate blood pressure and the immune system and modulate allergic and inflammatory responses. Some types of eicosanoids are highly inflammatory and linked to numerous health disorders—including hypertension—whereas others are anti-inflammatory and actually boost your immune system. The good news is that we can manipulate the type of eicosanoids formed in our bodies simply by changing what we eat. Omega-3 fats help us produce more of the good, anti-inflammatory kind and less of the disease-causing variety.

Boosting omega-3 fatty acid intake is not an easy task. Only a few sources provide the special plant omega-3 fat ALA, including English walnuts, some leafy greens, soy, grapeseed and canola oils, and flaxseed (the last of these is the richest plant source of ALA). Because plant-based omega-3s are so hard to find, most of the science backing the blood-pressure-lowering benefits of omega-3 uses the long-chain marine omega-3s, which can be consumed in two ways: by eating fatty types of fish and from fish oil pills.

Bringing Down Pressure and Cardiovascular Disease Risk with Omega-3 Fats

A growing body of scientific evidence supports the effectiveness of omega-3 fats in lowering blood pressure. A meta-analysis of randomized controlled trials of the effect of fish oil supplementation on blood pressure values, published in the *Journal of Hypertension*, showed that taking 3.7 grams of fish oil per day yielded a small but noteworthy decline in blood pressure of 2.1/1.6 mm Hg. (People with already diagnosed high blood pressure showed a greater decrease in pressure of 4/3 mm Hg.)[13] This may seem like an insignificant drop, but the authors noted that a reduction in blood pressure of just 5 mm Hg could prevent one-third of strokes and one-fifth of heart attacks in Western society—so fish oil can do a lot to nudge you in the right direction.

How Does Fish Oil Lower Blood Pressure?

Fish oil fights heart disease and promotes a meaningful drop in blood pressure in multiple ways. Read on to learn about several biological mechanisms responsible for the favorable effect of omega-3 fish fat on the arteries.

Method of attack #1: You may have heard the term "hardening of the arteries," which refers to a gradual loss of elasticity in the blood vessels that occurs with age and disease. This increasing arterial stiffness contributes to rising blood pressure, and taxes the heart by making it work harder to circulate blood. Fish oil makes stiff arteries more elastic. A recent systematic review of thirty-eight randomized controlled trials, published in the *American Journal of Clinical Nutrition*, showed that regular fish oil supplementation was able to reduce arterial stiffness, with the most efficacious daily dose estimated to be approximately 1 gram per day of combined EPA and DHA (540 mg of EPA and 360 mg of DHA).[14]

Method of attack #2: As you know, people with high blood pressure suffer from endothelial dysfunction, which occurs when the cells of the endothelium are inflamed and fail to produce enough of the potent vessel dilator nitric oxide. Well, it turns out that omega-3 fish fat makes your dysfunctional endothelium much more functional. A recent meta-analysis of sixteen randomized clinical trials showed that omega-3 fish oil supplementation (at dosages ranging from 0.5 to 4.5 grams/day) had a protective effect on the inner arterial wall, boosting production of nitric oxide and thereby lowering blood pressure.[15]

Method of attack #3: When it comes to fat, you truly are what you eat. The long-chain fatty acids EPA and DHA actually incorporate themselves into the walls of your red blood cells, making the cell walls more fluid and flexible. This allows them to squeeze down into the body's tiny capillaries more easily, transporting oxygen to all tissues of the body. Fish oil also effectively inhibits the ability of platelets to stick together, which thins the blood and reduces the likelihood of a fatal blood clot leading to a heart attack or stroke.[16] (Although thinning the blood will not affect your blood pressure per se, you are at increased risk of heart attack and stroke by virtue of your elevated pressure, so lessening your blood's tendency to clot is a wise preventative measure.)

Method of attack #4: As you have learned, fish oil lowers inflammation in the arteries by inhibiting the overproduction of inflammatory compounds your body produces when you consume omega-6 fats. According to a Finnish study of nearly fourteen hundred healthy, middle-aged men, as blood levels of EPA and DHA increased, levels of C-reactive protein (a blood marker of chronic inflammation) decreased.[17] (Note that high blood omega-3 content is a reflection of fish or fish oil consumption.)

Method of attack #5: Eating a daily fish meal can help you lose weight *and* millimeters of mercury. That was the takeaway message from an Australian study of sixty-three overweight men and women with high blood pressure. Researchers placed subjects on four different diets for a period of twelve weeks: a weight maintenance diet, a weight maintenance diet including a daily fish meal, a calorie-restricted diet, and a calorie-restricted diet including a daily fish meal. There was no change in body weight in the two groups following the weight maintenance diets, while the calorie-restriction groups both lost an average of twelve pounds—illustrating that when it comes to weight loss, it's all about calorie intake. So it should come as no surprise that compared with the control groups, the weight loss diet groups reduced their systolic and diastolic blood pressure values by 5.5/1.3 mm Hg. But beyond weight loss, the study showed that fish intake in and of itself has beneficial effects on blood pressure. The fish-eating weight maintenance group lowered their blood pressure by 6.0/3.0 mm Hg without losing any weight. And the fish-eating calorie-controlled group cut systolic and diastolic blood pressure by a phenomenal 13/9 mm Hg.[18] This proves that the best way to power down the pressure is by combining fish intake with a calorie-restricted diet.

You should also know that the benefits of omega-3 fats extend well beyond blood pressure management. They can help lower your triglyceride levels as well as prevent arrhythmias (abnormalities in the electrical activity of the heart).

Fish, Supplements, or Both?

Obtaining marine omega-3s solely from fish oil capsules may not have the same effect as eating the fish itself. Supplements have proven to be effective in reducing blood pressure, but we don't know whether they provide you with the additional benefits of actually eating fish. For example, we know from the famed INTER-MAP study, which analyzed eating habits from seventeen population samples in four countries (China, Japan, the United Kingdom, and the United States), that routine fish meals lower blood pressure.[19] Eating fish also provides you with the added benefits of preventing heart disease and increasing longevity. This is why I recommend that you not only strive for at least two fatty fish meals per week (plus a daily source of plant omega-3 fat, ALA) but also pop a daily supplement of 1–2 grams of fish oil.

Purity Issues with OTC Supplements

Over-the-counter fish oil pills are widely available, but what you see on the label may not be exactly what you are putting in your mouth. The Food and Drug Administration (FDA) regulates dietary supplements as a category of food and not as drugs, which means they are not subject to strict regulations. The supplement makers must list their ingredients, but that does not necessarily guarantee safety or the quality of the product. So the supplement industry is pretty much left to self-regulation, resulting in questionable product quality, consistency, potency, and purity. There may well be substandard fish oil pills on your drugstore shelf, so prescription fish oil pills are a good option. Lovaza, formerly known as Omacor, is a brand-name prescription fish oil supplement and is guaranteed by the FDA to be safe, to be high-quality, to be free of contaminants and impurities, and to contain exactly what the label says. One Lovaza capsule provides approximately 900 mg of mixed EPA and DHA omega-3 fatty acids. Talk to your doctor about taking a Lovaza pill daily to hit your omega-3 target. (You should know that doctors are advised by the Food and Drug Administration to prescribe Lovaza only for patients with highly elevated levels of triglycerides in their bloodstream and not for treating high blood pressure.)

A SHOT OF VEGETABLE JUICE A DAY KEEPS
BLOOD PRESSURE AT BAY

Next we'll see why a daily glass of low-sodium vegetable juice is one of the simplest ways to help you get in all the blood-pressure-battling nutrients required by the Blood Pressure Down plan.

Vegetable juice is technically a food, but in the Blood Pressure Down plan we're looking at it as a dietary supplement, intended to provide nutrients that may be missing from the diet or may not be consumed in a sufficient enough quantity to meet the person's needs. As we discussed in Chapter Six, reaching your daily potassium prescription of 4,700 mg per day is a tall order for many people. To help you achieve this goal, the Blood Pressure Down plan includes a daily shot of vegetable juice, which will pump up your potassium count in just a few delicious gulps.

> One glass of low-sodium vegetable juice provides you with a megadose of potassium, the blood-pressure-lowering mineral superstar: 900 mg in just 8 ounces, and all that for just 50 calories.

SUPPLEMENT CAUTION

Some of the supplements recommended in the Blood Pressure Down plan can have adverse side effects, particularly fish oil. After taking fish oil supplements, some people experience an unpleasant sensation sometimes called "fish burp," which is exactly what it sounds like. (Fish burps are not harmful to you, unless you are on your first date!) On a more serious note, there are concerns that excessive amounts of DHA and EPA could interfere with blood clotting, particularly in patients taking blood-thinning medications such as aspirin, warfarin, or clopidogrel. This prompted the AHA to issue a warning that taking more than 3 grams of omega-3 fish oil a day from capsules could cause excessive bleeding in some peo-

HOW TO KILL OFF YOUR LAB ANIMAL

What would happen if you fed your laboratory animals too much sodium and too little potassium? Researchers found that a long-term excess of sodium and deficit of potassium in an animal's body would result in high blood pressure and tissue damage—just like in our own bodies. Here are the specific effects:

- **Arteries:** high blood pressure, enlargement of smooth muscle (constrictor) cells, endothelial dysfunction, hardening and stiffening of arteries
- **Heart:** heart attack, heart enlargement, heart failure
- **Brain:** stroke
- **Kidneys:** sodium retention, potassium deficit, kidney disease
- **Metabolism and other effects:** insulin resistance, glucose intolerance, increase in action of the sympathetic nervous system

The takeaway? These animal studies underscore just how bad a sodium/potassium imbalance is for *anyone's* health (human or our four-legged friends).

Sources: Adrogué HJ, Madias NE. Sodium and potassium in the pathogenesis of hypertension. *New Eng J Med* 2007;356(19):1966–1978; Allyn M. Salt and hypertension lessons from animal models that relate to human hypertension: session II—animal models. *Hypertens* 1991;17:159–160.

ple. If you are taking these or other medications, check with your doctor about possible drug interactions.

While we're on the subject of dietary supplements, you should know that several herbal remedies on the market have been shown to *increase* blood pressure, and so obviously you should avoid taking these. The big ones to avoid are St. John's wort, ephedra (ma huang), yohimbe, and licorice.[20]

FILLING THE PRESCRIPTION

The best approach to lowering blood pressure with lifestyle changes is to choose a low-sodium diet filled with plenty of colorful fruits and vegetables, some fat-free dairy, and two fish meals a week. Pair the food with a daily glass of red wine and the supplementation program outlined in this chapter and you'll be eating your way to better health and lower blood pressure.

The three most powerful blood-pressure-lowering lifestyle strategies known to humankind are diet, exercise, and stress management. Note that food is just one part of this equation. This brings us to the final step in the Blood Pressure Down plan: exercise and stress management. So get your sneakers on and get ready to walk off that stress and walk down that pressure!

13

Step 10: Exercise

℞ Walk, Jog, Swim, or Cycle for Thirty Minutes Every Day (and Relax
for Ten)

Why do virtually all major health agencies throughout the world
advocate regular exercise as cornerstone therapy for the prevention,
treatment, and control of high blood pressure? Perhaps it's because
couch potatoes have a 50 percent greater risk of developing high
blood pressure.[1] Or maybe it's because of the overwhelming scientific evidence that just a little bit of moderate exercise—taken on
a daily basis—is medicinal magic for getting blood pressure numbers down to a healthy level. Indeed, exercise is the best medicine
both for keeping the arteries wide and flexible and for diffusing
stress, which is a destructive, blood-pressure-raising enemy. In our
tenth and final Blood Pressure Down step, we move away from the
kitchen and out to the grass, sidewalk, gym, or pool, to focus on
moving the body and calming the mind—two wonderfully safe and
incredibly effective lifestyle measures for easing the pressure and
getting your numbers where you want them to be. So lace up your
walking shoes, get out your yoga mat, and prepare to exercise and
relax your blood pressure down!

EXERCISE: MOTHER NATURE'S NATURAL
BLOOD PRESSURE MEDICINE

The simple act of putting on your sneakers and taking a thirty-minute walk every day is as effective in lowering your millimeters of mercury as some prescription drugs. Habitual aerobic exercise (sometimes called *cardio*) such as walking, swimming, and biking lowers blood pressure between 5 and 10 mm Hg.[2] Recall that what may seem like an insignificant decrease of just 2 mm Hg in both the top (systolic) and bottom (diastolic) numbers can cut risk of stroke by

MOVING MORE FIGHTS "SITTING DISEASE"

Being a couch potato is even worse for your arteries than you might think. New research has shown that long periods of sitting are extremely detrimental to your health, increasing your risk of disease no matter how active or fit a person you are. British scientists linked prolonged periods of sitting (at a computer, watching television, or doing anything sedentary) to a greater likelihood of developing diabetes, cardiovascular disease, breast and colon cancer, and obesity. Piggybacking on this finding, Australian researchers reported that each average daily hour spent watching TV is linked to an 18 percent increase in the risk of death from heart disease. How could sitting still harm the arteries, you might wonder? Scientists have investigated just this question, and the results are frightening. Inactivity actually causes dangerous adaptive structural changes within the circulatory system: your arteries shrink in size and the arterial walls get thicker. This is bad news for your blood pressure, as small, thick, inflexible arteries are the hallmark of high blood pressure, cardiovascular disease, and premature death.

Sources: Owen N, Bauman A, Brown W. Too much sitting: a novel and important predictor of chronic disease risk? *Br J Sport Med* 2009;43(2):81–83; Dunstan, DW, Barr ELM, Healy GN, et al. Television viewing time and mortality: the Australian Diabetes, Obesity and Lifestyle study (AusDiab). *Circulation* 2010;121:384–391; Thijssen DHJ, Green DJ, Hopman MTE. Blood vessel remodeling and physical inactivity in humans. *J Appl Physiol* 2011;111:1836–1845.

14 and 17 percent and risk of a heart attack by 9 and 6 percent![3] Pretty remarkable results for simply taking a daily stroll in the park. So let's take a closer look at what the research tells us about how much, how often, and what kind of exercise is best for attaining these phenomenal results.

A LITTLE CARDIO CUTS BLOOD PRESSURE NUMBERS

Regular aerobic exercise is an effective treatment for diagnosed high blood pressure and lowers your risk of developing high blood pressure in the first place.[4] That's the takeaway message from the ample research that supports the positive effect of exercise on blood pressure.

Exercise Works Regardless of Your Current Fitness Level or Body Weight

If you are currently sedentary and decide to take up exercise, it will truly do wonders for your blood pressure numbers. A meta-analysis published in the prestigious journal *Annals of Internal Medicine* compiled data from fifty-four randomized clinical trials with 2,419 participants to determine the effects of regular aerobic exercise on blood pressure.[5] The results? A regular exercise program has an impressive blood-pressure-lowering effect in previously sedentary individuals, with reductions in both systolic and diastolic blood pressure of 4/3 mm Hg. Blood pressure dropped in virtually everyone—people with high blood pressure and those with normal blood pressure, overweight people and normal-weight people, and blacks, whites, and Asians. It is important to note that aerobic exercise has been shown to lower blood pressure in individuals with high blood pressure who have a normal body weight, allowing scientists to conclude that exercise itself results in blood pressure reductions, independent of weight loss.

In another meta-analysis of forty-four randomized controlled intervention trials involving nearly three thousand participants, the results were equally supportive of the blood-pressure-lowering effect of exercise. When sedentary people began to exercise (mainly walking, jogging, running, or cycling) for an average of forty minutes three times per week, their average blood pressure after 16 weeks had declined by 3/2 mm Hg in people with normal blood pressure and an amazing 7/6 mm Hg in those with high blood pressure.[6]

What Do Experts Recommend as the Optimal Exercise Prescription?

American College of Sports Medicine (ACSM). The ACSM is the premier governing body on all things related to exercise. They recommend a program of primarily aerobic exercise as an integral component of the lifestyle prescription for the prevention, treatment, and control of high blood pressure.[7] For those individuals with diagnosed high blood pressure, they prescribe the following exercise plan:

> *Frequency:* on most, preferably all, days of the week
> *Intensity:* moderate
> *Time:* at least thirty minutes of physical activity (this can be accomplished by getting in your exercise all at once for at least thirty minutes or via multiple bouts per day, as long as your exercise time totals thirty minutes or more)
> *Type:* primarily endurance physical activity, such as walking, jogging, biking, or swimming, supplemented by strength training

U.S. Department of Health and Human Services. The recommendations in the 2008 Department of Health and Human Services (DHHS) *Physical Activity Guidelines Advisory Committee Report* are consistent with the ACSM guidelines.[8] The DHHS concluded that both aerobic exercise and resistance exercise reduce blood pressure, but the evidence backing aerobic exercise is much more substantial. According to the report, the following exercise prescription yields significant blood pressure reduction in those with high blood pressure:

Frequency: three to five times per week

Intensity: moderate to high intensity

Time: forty minutes of aerobic exercise training per day

Type: twelve miles per week of walking or jogging (note that for weight loss of 5 percent or more, the DHHS recommends greater amounts of physical activity, equivalent to walking about forty-five minutes per day at four miles per hour, walking about seventy minutes per day at three miles per hour, or jogging twenty-two minutes per day at six miles per hour)

GOT PREHYPERTENSION? A LITTLE EXERCISE GETS YOUR NUMBERS DOWN

No marathons required here! Just three short ten-minute walking sessions (adding up to thirty minutes a day) are enough to make a meaningful dent in your prehypertensive numbers. Researchers found that thirty minutes of accumulated walking got systolic pressure down a whopping 4 mm Hg in twenty prehypertensive subjects. This is good news for you if you can't fathom the idea of a traditional thirty-minute workout every day. Just walking to and from work plus a ten-minute stroll with the dog is all you need. And while 4 mm Hg may not seem like much, you know by now that every millimeter counts. A 3 mm Hg reduction in systolic blood pressure can dramatically cut your odds of dying young and gives you an 8 percent lower chance of a stroke and 5 percent lower odds of a heart attack.

Sources: Park S, Rink LD, Wallace JP. Accumulation of physical activity: blood pressure reduction between 10-min walking sessions. *J Hum Hypertens* 2008;22:475–482; Chobanian AV, Bakris GL, Black HR, et al. The seventh report of the Joint National Committee on Prevention, Detection, Evaluation, and Treatment of High Blood Pressure: the JNC 7 report. *JAMA* 2003;289(19):2560–2571.

Calories Well Spent: The Blood Pressure Down Exercise Prescription

Well, now you know what the exercise experts recommend to get your blood pressure down. So let's take what they suggest and mold it into a doable plan *for you*. My patients often ask me, "What's the best exercise?" and my response is invariably, "Any exercise that you will *do*!" Sticking with an exercise is key, so the one indisputable aspect of the optimal exercise plan for you is that it be sustainable. Take what you will from the exercise prescription below and know that getting in *some form* of exercise every day is invaluable medicine for keeping your pressure and arteries healthy.

> *Frequency:* on most, preferably all, days of the week
> *Intensity:* mild to moderate
> *Time:* at least thirty minutes of continuous or accumulated aerobic (cardio) exercise per day
> *Type:* primarily endurance physical activity, such as walking, jogging, biking, or swimming, supplemented by strength training two days a week

Walking Works—but So Does Swimming

As you can see, the ideal exercise prescription for lowering blood pressure involves a daily bout of cardio exercise. Walking is one of the safest, simplest, and most inexpensive blood-pressure-improvement strategies you can adopt to complete your daily attack on your pressure. However, if you prefer swimming, you should know that a recent study from the Cardiovascular Aging Research Laboratory at the University of Texas has some great news.[9] Forty-three hypertensive or prehypertensive men and women between the ages of fifty and eighty were divided into a swimming exercise group and a control group. For twelve weeks, the swimmers swam fifteen to twenty minutes at a fairly low intensity, three to four days a week. The results were nothing short of phenomenal. The swimmers' systolic blood pressure dropped from an average of 131 mm Hg to 122 mm Hg (plus a 4 mm drop in diastolic pressure). What's more, swimming produced a 21 percent increase in "carotid artery compliance," a measure of the elasticity and flexibility of the central artery going from the heart to the brain.

How Hard Is Too Hard?

It doesn't take a herculean effort to get those millimeters down with exercise. In fact, if exercising hard is not your cup of tea, you should know that even light exercise can do wonders for your blood pressure control.[10] One group of researchers looked at the blood pressure benefits of both high- and low-intensity exercise and found

STRONG MEN (WITH HYPERTENSION) LIVE LONGER

Clearly a little cardio exercise, performed on most days of the week, prevents and treats high blood pressure and cuts risk of premature mortality in people with diagnosed high blood pressure. But what about strength training? If you have been diagnosed with high blood pressure, is there any benefit to pumping iron—and is it safe? A recent eighteen-year study of more than fifteen hundred middle-aged men with hypertension, published in the *Journal of the American College of Cardiology*, found that the men with the greatest muscular strength had a 41 percent lower risk of premature death than their weaker counterparts. The researchers concluded that the simple act of lifting weights can protect against an early demise, particularly among those with high blood pressure. The moral of the story: get to the gym at least twice per week and lift weights to live longer and stronger. (To lower blood pressure most effectively, spend more of your workout time on cardio.) One caveat: be careful not to strain. Perform more repetitions at lighter weights to prevent your blood pressure from temporarily spiking.

Source: Artero EG, Lee D-C, Ruiz JR, et al. A prospective study of muscular strength and all-cause mortality in men with hypertension. *J Am Coll Cardiol* 2011;57(18):1831–1837.

that ten weeks of varied aerobic exercise training at either high or low intensity reduced blood pressure in a similar manner, suggesting that intensity is not a major factor in lowering blood pressure. The authors concluded that frequency, time, and type of exercise are more important than how hard you're working out.[11]

EXERCISE SAFELY

If exercise has not routinely been part of your lifestyle, *make sure you get the go-ahead from your physician before beginning your exercise program.* Here are some important tips for exercising safely:

1. If you are taking prescription medications for high blood pressure, such as beta-blockers or ACE inhibitors, you should know that they can alter your blood pressure and heart rate response to exercise. Discuss these side effects with your personal physician.

2. Warm up for at least five minutes to reduce the chances of a sharp and sudden rise in blood pressure. A slow walk before you begin your workout is ideal to get the blood flowing and to help your body adjust to the stress of exercise.

3. Allow for an adequate cool-down period to help transition the body to its pre-exercise state and prevent dizziness and fainting, which could be caused by blood pooling in the legs.

4. Perform an easy stretching routine after your cardio. It may not feel like a workout, but this is a segment of your exercise routine that should not be omitted. Stretching after your muscles are all warmed up will help increase your flexibility, and flexibility is one category of physical fitness that severely declines with age.

5. Remember to stay hydrated and dress for the elements! Drink water before, during, and after your workout.

Cold weather requires breathable layers of clothing and a hat (approximately 30 percent of body heat is lost from the head). Warm and humid weather requires light, breathable clothing as well as a hat to protect skin against damage from the sun. If the outdoor weather is severe—either extremely cold or hot and humid or there is lightning—exercise indoors.

6. Maintain normal breathing during exercise, especially during strength training. The goal is to prevent the Valsava effect, a forced expiration of air with your trachea closed. This occurs when you hold your breath on exertion—which causes a steep rise in blood pressure.

7. Build your exercise routine gradually and avoid the "weekend warrior" mentality. Remember, consistency is more important than intensity!

8. If you have chest pains, feel light-headed or dizzy, or experience severe shortness of breath or pain, stop exercising and immediately call your physician.

DEFUSING STRESS AND LOWERING BLOOD PRESSURE

Keep in mind that chronic stress is a leading cause of high blood pressure and is highly damaging to the body. Yes, stress will always be a part of daily life. But when excessive stress over an extended period of time is combined with poor coping strategies, it can lead to disease and even death. For example, multiple large-scale studies have shown that individuals who report high levels of mental stress have nearly twice the risk of fatal strokes as those with low stress levels.[12,13]

It's important to note that people who report *experiencing* more stress don't necessarily *have* more stress in their lives. In most cases, less stressed people have similar stresses but are able to release their stress in a healthy manner, rather than internalizing it. Learning how to defuse your own body's stress response is vital medicine for bringing your blood pressure down and preventing other adverse health effects. The good news is that stress relief comes in many forms, and surely at least one of these techniques will be right for you. Read on and learn how easy it is to put a damper on your stress response—a simple and effective first line of defense against the silent killer hypertension, and the final series of exercises in the Blood Pressure Down plan.

When Stress Is Harmful

Even a small stressor can enlist the body's fight-or-flight response. When confronted by stress, your brain signals your adrenal glands, which sit on top of your kidneys, to release the stress hormones cortisol and adrenaline to help you cope. You may have experienced these effects before you have to make a big presentation or when you narrowly avoid a fender bender. These stress hormones produce increased heart rate, dilation of the pupils, sweating, blood vessel constriction, and other reactions regulated by the sympathetic nervous system. Even a small stress response causes your blood vessels to constrict. Research is just beginning to unlock the complex relationship between chronic stress and the development of high blood pressure and other cardiovascular diseases, but the good news is that practicing simple relaxation strategies can calm your physiology, destress your mind, and quickly reverse the fight-or-flight response to prevent the deleterious effects of chronic stress on your arteries. Getting in your daily bout of cardio exercise is one perfect outlet for stress—it provides distraction from daily troubles as well as enhances the body's ability to deal with stress. In addition to your workout, your arteries will benefit from practicing other types of stress-busting quick relief strategies, the relaxation therapies.

Letting Off Steam with Exercises That Induce Relaxation

Relaxation therapy is the antidote to the stress response. Practicing relaxation techniques has been shown to tame the sympathetic

DEEP SLEEP KEEPS PRESSURE NORMAL

Sleep is important for maintaining good health. But it's not just how *much* you sleep that matters—*how* you sleep counts, too.

As you probably know, human sleep is cyclical and is divided into REM (rapid eye movement) sleep and non-REM sleep. REM is the sleep stage where you dream and is the last stage in the cycle. Non-REM sleep is further divided into four stages, each of which can last from five to fifteen minutes. Typically we begin at stage 1 and go through all four non-REM stages, switch to REM sleep, and then begin the cycle again. Stage 1 is a light sleep with eye and body movements slowed. During stage 2, a slightly deeper sleep, your brain waves begin to slow as well (50 percent of your sleep time occurs in this stage). Stages 3 and 4 are known as slow-wave deep sleep and are the most crucial stages for restorative health.

New research has shown that getting enough deep, slow-wave sleep is important for maintaining a healthy blood pressure. In a study of eight hundred men with normal blood pressure, men with the lowest levels of slow-wave sleep (stages 3 and 4) had an 80 percent greater risk of developing high blood pressure over the three-and-a-half-year study period compared to the good sleepers. How does one get a better night's sleep? Utilize the natural relaxation exercises described in this chapter in lieu of sedative medications, which actually decrease the amount of slow-wave sleep in the sleep cycle.

In addition, sleep apnea—characterized by snoring and frequent pauses in breathing during sleep—is also associated with high blood pressure. Treating sleep apnea with lifestyle changes such as weight loss and/or a continuous positive airway pressure (CPAP) machine has been proven to improve blood pressure.

Source: Fung MM, Peters K, Redline S, et al. Decreased slow wave sleep increases risk of developing hypertension in elderly men. *Hypertens* 2011;58:596–603.

nervous system and lead to a reduction in blood pressure. So as part of the Blood Pressure Down plan, you are going to learn and practice stress-reduction exercises. This is the best "medicine" for ameliorating the harmful effects of stress, calming your body and your mind. (Stress management is so effective that the Canadian government has listed it as part of its lifestyle therapeutic approach for individuals with hypertension.)[14]

Relaxation lifestyle treatments fall under four general categories:

1. Physical techniques such as yoga, breathing exercises, and progressive muscle relaxation
2. Biofeedback, a method that uses the mind to control involuntary bodily functions such as blood pressure
3. Autogenic training relaxation techniques, which teach your body to respond to verbal cues to relax and control breathing
4. Cognitive-behavioral therapy, such as guided imagery, talk therapy, and meditation

Do Relaxation Therapies Work?

Researchers in the United Kingdom performed a meta-analysis of twenty-five randomized controlled trials, involving nearly twelve hundred participants, to investigate whether or not different types of relaxation therapy are effective in lowering pressure.[15] They found that a regular program of relaxation therapy results in a drop in blood pressure of 6/4 mm Hg, and that progressive muscle relaxation, biofeedback, and cognitive-behavioral therapies were the types most likely to be effective.

Yoga Techniques Soothe Psychological Stress and Lower Pressure

Yoga is mind-body therapy that has been shown to impart peace of mind as well as a notable drop in blood pressure. In one Indian study, scientists randomly assigned 60 men and women with high blood pressure to one of three groups: daily fast-paced breathing exercises; daily slow-breathing yoga exercises; and a control group.[16] At the end of the three-month study period, the group

PETS BEAT DRUGS FOR BLUNTING STRESS-INDUCED PRESSURE

Imagine this: you are in a high-stress profession and have high blood pressure, for which you are taking an ACE inhibitor (lisinopril). You decide to get a dog or cat, and when you take your blood pressure at home, you notice that it has dropped an additional 10 mm Hg compared to the pre-pet days. Sound too good to be true? This phenomenon is exactly what investigators proved in a study of forty-eight stressed-out individuals with high blood pressure.

Subjects were divided into two groups: one group was assigned a pet (a cat or dog, depending on personal preference) in addition to their 20 mg/day of lisinopril, while the control group simply took the lisinopril. After six months, the pet owners had an average blood pressure of 131/92 compared to 141/100 in the control group, and the renin activity in their blood was significantly lower too—recall that high renin activity in the blood triggers high pressure. The authors concluded that pets have a greater calming influence on the sympathetic nervous system than ACE inhibitor therapy alone. After all, pets are nonjudgmental and always accepting of their owners, making them ideal candidates for enhancing lives—and providing health benefits.

Source: Allen K, Shykoff BE, Izzo JL. Pet ownership, but not inhibitor therapy, blunts home blood pressure responses to mental stress. *Hypertens* 2001;38:815–820.

practicing the slow-breathing yoga techniques showed miraculous pressure responses, cutting their numbers by about 10 mm Hg systolic and 7 mm Hg diastolic. The scientists concluded that simple slow-breathing yoga therapy is an effective tool for dramatically reducing blood pressure and could even eliminate the need for prescription medications to control the disease.

A recent nursing journal review of evidence-based research also confirmed that yoga does indeed reduce those millimeters of mercury.[17] In this review, yoga therapy consisted of *asanas* (body postures) in combination with *pranayama* (breathing exercises). Eight of the nine studies under review demonstrated that yoga lowers blood pressure through its ability to modulate the body's physiology. Yoga can favorably affect the body's autonomic nervous system—the part of the nervous system that regulates involuntary physiological functions, the ones that are normally not under our conscious control, such as heart and breathing rates. Note that the practice of yoga breathing exercises alone, without the addition of physical postures, also showed significant blood pressure benefits.

Transcendental Meditation Curbs Blood Pressure and Cuts Risk of Early Death

Transcendental meditation is one of the most widely practiced and researched meditation techniques. It is based on the teachings of the Maharishi Mahesh Yogi and involves the repetition of a sound or mantra, practiced for twenty minutes twice per day. The mantra repetition can be spoken or chanted, whispered, or silent (you simply think the mantra).

Transcendental meditation has proven to be an effective tool in the fight against high blood pressure.[18] A recent meta-analysis of well-designed randomized controlled clinical trials compared the stress- and blood-pressure-reducing effects of various stress reduction approaches,[19] including biofeedback, relaxation-assisted biofeedback, progressive muscle relaxation, stress management training, and transcendental meditation. The results? Transcendental mediation was best for promoting a significant drop in blood pressure (5.0/2.8 mm Hg). Another study, published in the *American Journal of Cardiology*, analyzed data from more than two hundred older patients with high blood pressure, followed for an average of eighteen years. The results were quite spectacular: the subjects who practiced transcendental meditation cut their risk of death from heart disease by 30 percent and their risk of death from cancer in half.[20] Clearly, transcendental meditation heals the mind and body, and helps you live longer.

Slow Breathing Combined with Meditation Calms the Numbers

Slow breathing exercises (six cycles of breath per minute, or one deep breath in and out lasting ten seconds, for several minutes), have been shown to result in a drop in blood pressure numbers in people with high blood pressure.[21] And combining slow breathing with mindful meditation appears to be a one-two punch against pressure. A randomized controlled trial of fifty-two people with high blood pressure who were not taking prescription medication found that subjects who underwent eight weeks of contemplative meditation/breathing exercise treatment lowered their blood pressure a substantial amount—their blood pressure reaction under a heavy mental stress load was a full 11 mm Hg lower than the control group.[22]

TEN SIMPLE STRESS-BUSTERS

Now that you know that your uncontrolled high stress lifestyle is a dangerous force that elevates your pressure, you understand the importance of practicing healthful stress management to tame the mercury readings. Here are ten ways to defuse the stress bomb, calming your body, your mind, and your numbers:

1. **Walk, run, swim, or cycle.** Exercise dissipates the stress hormones that raise your pressure.
2. **Get a good night's sleep.** As you learned, lack of sleep, especially deep-wave sleep, contributes to raising pressure.
3. **Get a pet.** If you like animals, get one and bask in its unconditional love. (Petting animals has been shown to reduce the stress hormone cortisol.)
4. **Try tai chi.** Tai chi is a type of exercise derived from Chinese martial arts. The focus is on slow, rhythmic movements, used to create a state of mental clarity and well-being.
5. **Try yoga.** Yoga is a popular ancient spiritual art form rooted in Indian culture. Yoga involves breathing exercises as well as movement through a series of postures (asanas).

---

6. **Try meditation.** Another ancient technique proven to quiet the mind, meditation slows brain waves and cuts your pressure.

7. **Try guided imagery.** Guided imagery involves tapping into happy memories and using the mind to create visual scenes of peaceful places where you concentrate on the scene to make it seem as if you are really there. (See the Quick Guided Imagery Exercise Guidelines in Appendix 1.)

8. **Listen to calming music.** Peaceful music can impact the subconscious, slowing brain waves and leading to relaxed states.

9. **Try relaxation breathing.** Try closing your eyes and focusing solely on your breath. Breathe very deeply and aim to gradually slow down to six cycles per minute. (Normal breathing is about twelve breaths per minute.) Deep breathing can effectively alter the activity of the nervous system, lowering your heart rate and blood pressure.

10. **Do your best.** The adage "Do your best and leave the rest" will help you to make the most of stressful situations over which you have little or no control. It is usually your *reaction* to a situation, not the situation itself, that is the primary cause of stress.

HOW EXERCISE AND STRESS MANAGEMENT CUT BLOOD PRESSURE NUMBERS

Different types of exercise are effective at lowering blood pressure. Let's see why exercise is the best medicine for keeping your arteries healthy and your blood pressure down.

Method of attack #1: People with high blood pressure have peripheral vascular resistance, which (as you may remember from Chapter Two) means that the network of tiny arteries that feed the body's tissues are too resistant to blood flow. When you exercise, your body experiences a robust increase in blood flow through your arteries to your active skeletal muscles. Over time, the repeated increase diminishes systemic vascular resistance and reduces blood pressure.

Method of attack #2: Bumping up the intensity of your workouts is beneficial for your blood vessels because it increases what is termed "shear stress"—the speed of blood flowing through the blood vessels. Increasing shear stress for an extended period, such as when you take a brisk walk, prompts the cells lining your arteries to increase production of their own anti-inflammatory chemicals, as well as release more chemical relaxers such as nitric oxide and inhibit the production of chemical tighteners. Brazilian researchers, for example, found that six months of moderate-intensity exercise training (stationary bicycling for sixty minutes, three days a week) was enough to increase nitric oxide level by an incredible 60 percent in eleven sedentary, postmenopausal women with diagnosed high blood pressure.[23] All of this heals damaged arteries, helps prevent clogging, and lessens the chance of a heart attack or stroke. Exercise is also effective medicine for reversing arterial

INTERVAL TRAINING BEATS CONTINUOUS EXERCISE FOR BLOOD PRESSURE BENEFITS

Interval exercise training, where you alternate between high and low intensities during your workout, may be just what it takes to relax the arteries. Higher-intensity training subjects your arteries to greater shear stress, and arteries adapt to this stress by becoming less stiff and more flexible. A recent study found that interval training was superior to continuous exercise training for reducing arterial stiffness in individuals with high blood pressure.

Source: Guimarães GV, Ciolac EG, Carvalho VO, et al. Effects of continuous vs. interval exercise training on blood pressure and arterial stiffness in treated hypertension. *Hypertens Res* 2010;33:627–632.

stiffening—the hallmark of an aging artery, which is much more pronounced in people with high blood pressure.[24]

Method of attack #3: As we discussed in Chapter Nine, oxidative stress leads to inflammation and accelerated arterial damage. People with high blood pressure have higher levels of oxidative stress, which impacts blood pressure through an intricate mechanism of blood vessel constriction. Oxidative stress also causes endothelial dysfunction, which results from the insufficient production and dispersal of nitric oxide. Exercise mends the injured endothelium by activating the body's natural repair systems.[25] An increase in production of homegrown antioxidants as well as nitric oxide helps your body to lower dangerous levels of cellular oxidative stress and soothe inflammation.

Method of attack #4: Recall from Chapter Two that an elevation in blood pressure involves an overactive sympathetic nervous system and renin-angiotensin system. Regular exercise puts the brakes on these systems, leading to a relaxation of the arteries and subsequent drop in pressure.

Method of attack #5: Make no mistake about it: losing excess body fat is one of your most powerful weapons in the fight against high blood pressure. Being overweight makes your arteries more prone to becoming stiff and constricted. As you know by now, attaining a healthy body weight and losing body fat—especially belly fat—will greatly contribute to the reversal of your disease process. Becoming overweight is the result of routinely consuming too many calories combined with burning too few. A healthy rate of weight loss is attained when you create a calorie deficit—a situation where you consistently expend more calories than you consume. Exercising regularly will make it much easier for you to accomplish your weight-loss (and blood pressure) goals.

Method of attack #6: Is it true that some yogis in India and elsewhere can use their mind to control seemingly involuntary body functions such as heart rate and blood pressure? In a way, yes—the mind may just be your most powerful blood-pressure-lowering medication. The autonomic (involuntary) nervous system controls bodily functions that are largely below our level of consciousness, such as digestion, breathing rate, heart rate, and blood pressure. People with high blood pressure often have a defect in the autonomic nervous system's control of heart rate and blood pressure. Slow-breathing exercises have been proven to improve the autonomic nervous system's ability to control blood pressure, promoting a significant reduction in both systolic and diastolic pressures.[26] I urge you to take time every day to tap into your mind to calm your nerves, and in so doing, get your numbers where you need them to be—naturally.

TIPS FOR GETTING IN YOUR DAILY DOSE OF EXERCISE

- Make exercise a priority in your life. If you cast a positive light on exercise and acknowledge that it is the best medicine for healing your arteries, improving your joie de vivre, and especially for releasing harmful blood-pressure-raising stress, then you will be more likely to embrace this lifetime prescription.
- To ensure you stick with it, start slow. Maybe begin with just a walk around the block, and build up over time to your goal distance or duration.
- Set a target: choose a set distance and plan to walk, jog, cycle, or swim that distance and back, every day.
- Wear the right clothes and the right shoes. Don't forget to hydrate before and after you exercise, and remember to protect yourself against the elements.
- Exercise with a buddy or your dog if you prefer company; this may make the task more enjoyable for you.
- Purchase a portable music player and listen to your favorite tunes while you exercise off your stress.
- Walk indoors on a treadmill. Place it in front of the television and walk during your favorite show.

- Hire a personal trainer. If you pay for strength training, you will more likely go for your appointment.
- Join a gym and take classes that you might enjoy, such as group lap swimming, stepping, dance exercise, or cycling. (I personally like cycling classes. Forty-five minutes of "dancing" on a bike—at a level that I can accomplish—makes daily exercise a fun and doable treat for me.)
- Practice your deep breathing and/or mediation at a set time every day—perhaps right after work or at a time during your day when you know you have reached your limit. (I always practice deep breathing exercise when I am stressed out sitting in bumper-to-bumper traffic!)
- Purchase exercise clothes that make you feel good about yourself: fashions for yoga, running, swimming, or dance will help.

ANOTHER REMINDER: EXERCISE PRECAUTIONS

Make sure to get the go-ahead from your personal physician before you begin any exercise program. If you have been diagnosed with high blood pressure, you should ask your doctor for advice about an exercise routine that is right for you. If you are taking prescription medications for your blood pressure, depending on the class of drugs, you may need to take some extra exercise precautions:

- Thiazide diuretics increase loss of fluids and potassium. Make sure to get the recommended potassium intake daily (4,700 mg) and drink plenty of water.
- Beta-blockers lower your heart rate (pulse). When doing cardio exercises, do not be concerned if your

pulse fails to reach the target heart rate range (frequently posted on the wall in gyms). Never fear—you are still getting the phenomenal health benefits of exercise.

TAKE THE MEDICINE OF LIFE

Imagine a medication that could lower blood pressure, prevent diabetes, give you more energy, make it easier for you to lose weight, alleviate stress, and make you feel happy to be alive. That medicine exists, it's free, and it's called exercise! It should come as no surprise to those interested in following a natural health lifestyle that the key to controlling blood pressure is found not in a prescription bottle but instead in a pair of sneakers and a yoga mat. If lowering your blood pressure is not enough motivation to get you off the couch, try changing the focus to something that will motivate you. How about the simple act of making precious alone time for yourself to revel in your own thoughts every day? Getting your heart rate up, perhaps listening to your favorite music, and spending time alone with yourself will lift your spirits and make you feel good about yourself *instantly*. The well-being derived from a daily bout of exercise can be a powerful motivator for many people—even for those who dislike exercising.

I hope you have learned that the most efficient lifestyle approach to preventing and treating this silent killer is one that attacks the problem from several different directions, utilizing a multistep plan. Round out your healthy eating plan with a daily walk, a few minutes of mindful relaxation, and twice-weekly strength training sessions, and you have the secret to a healthy blood pressure reading and a long and happy life.

A Few Closing Words
from Dr. Janet

Persistent high blood pressure is a life-endangering situation. It puts a strain on your arteries, which can cause them to harden, become clogged, or weaken. This in turn increases your risk of heart disease and stroke. Sad to say, one in three Americans has this condition—making this a public health epidemic of great magnitude. The Institute of Medicine has deemed high blood pressure the "neglected disease" because it is easily detected and has a multitude of safe and low-cost interventions, both nonpharmacological and pharmacological, to rapidly bring blood pressure under control—and yet millions of Americans continue to live with and die from high blood pressure.[1] Health professionals and the public alike fail to translate this knowledge into practice—for what reason, I can't say.

I hope you have learned from this book that high blood pressure must no longer be neglected. It is the number one cause of stroke and a major cause of heart attacks. If left untreated, it can also lead to vision loss and kidney failure. High blood pressure kills more than 800,000 Americans each year, more than any other condition. Get your blood pressure down and you can prevent disease, disability, and premature death.

Relying on drug therapy to treat and prevent this global epidemic is akin to putting a Band-Aid on a gaping wound. Lifestyle modifications should serve as first-line therapy for the prevention and treatment of this disorder, with the specific changes outlined in this book as the foremost strategies for combatting this disease. I hope that with the Blood Pressure Down plan, you see how you can focus on the "can" rather than the "cannot." You've learned about all the delicious foods and activities that you will enjoy while making your health a priority.

Understand that when it comes to preventing and treating high blood pressure, it's strength in numbers—the more steps added together on a daily basis, the more powerful the blood-pressure-lowering effect of this combination lifestyle therapy plan. Many different foods, supplements, and exercise routines are individually effective in lowering blood pressure, but my patients and I have found that my Blood Pressure Down combination is the most potent nonpharmaceutical strategy for getting those numbers under control and promoting health.

It's not complicated. Many of the steps in the plan are basically plain old healthful eating, with no harmful side effects or expensive prescription medications. Most foods can be purchased at your local supermarket. Add in a few supplements, lose a few pounds, cut down on your sodium intake, and get some exercise in, and you have a safe and effective natural alternative (or adjunct) to prescription medication.

Ideally, it is best to get in all ten steps each day. However, nobody is perfect! Checking off as many as possible, as often as possible, will surely help you in your goal of getting your numbers where you want them to be. If you have already been diagnosed with an abnormally high blood pressure reading, take heart in knowing that you can take charge of your health and lower those numbers. With blood pressure, every millimeter counts.

Following these ten simple steps will surely add years to your life and life to your years. Good luck in following this plan—and sticking to it for the rest of your days. I sincerely hope that you are successful in getting, and keeping, your blood pressure down!

To your health,

Dr. Janet Brill

Appendixes

Appendix 1:

QUICK GUIDED IMAGERY EXERCISE GUIDELINES

 Time Required: 10 Minutes

What You Need

- Privacy
- Some quiet time
- A comfortable space
- Soothing music, if desired

Here's How

1. Remove yourself from the hectic world and find a comfortable spot where no one will bother you for at least ten minutes.
2. Unplug from the world—cell phone, computer, etc.
3. Begin by putting on soft, soothing music (if desired).
4. Close your eyes and begin to take long, deep breaths, focusing on your breathing (one breath cycle every ten seconds, five seconds in, five seconds out).
5. After a few minutes of deep breathing, you will have reached a more relaxed state. At this point, begin your

guided imagery journey by conjuring up in your mind a scene where you are at peace.

6. Personalize your journey by envisioning yourself in a place that has brought you serenity in your life. For some, this could be sailing on the crystal-clear waters of the Aegean. For others, it could be sitting in a comfy chair by a fire wrapped in a plush blanket, sipping hot chocolate, and watching the snow fall and the icicles melt.

7. As you imagine your scene, try to place yourself there physically and emotionally. Do you feel the ocean spray on your face and taste the salt water as you glide through the ocean? Can you hear the fire crackling, see the flames dancing, and smell the wood burning? Make your vision as real as possible by seeking to involve all your senses. What do you see, hear, feel, taste, and smell?

8. Stay in your world for as long as you like, far away from the stresses that are harming you. When you are ready to return to reality, prepare yourself by performing ten slow breath cycles, counting down from ten. When you reach one, open your eyes. You will return to the world feeling mentally refreshed, calmer, and ready to tackle life in a healthier manner.

Appendix 2:

TEN-STEP DAILY CHECKLIST

Day of the week: _____

Remember, the more steps you take today, the more potent the blood-pressure-lowering effect!

❑ ❑ ❑ **Banana** (and other high-potassium fruits)	❑ **Calories** (cut portion sizes and meet 1,800 or 2,000 total)
❑ ❑ **Nonfat plain yogurt** (with pumpkin)	❑ **Sodium** (1,500 mg maximum)
❑ ❑ **Soy** in place of animal protein	❑ **Dark chocolate** ❑ **Red wine** (1–2 glasses with a meal)
❑ ❑ ❑ ❑ ❑ **Spinach** (and other high-potassium veggies)	❑ **Supplements**: __Vitamin D$_3$ __ Fish oil __ CoQ$_{10}$ __ Low-sodium V8
	❑ **Exercises**: __Cardio __ Relaxation

Blood pressure (morning):_____ Blood pressure (afternoon):_____ Blood pressure (evening):_____

℞ **Potassium foods:** Eat foods totaling at least 4,700 mg of potassium every day.
Magnesium foods: Eat foods totaling at least 500 mg of magnesium every day.
Calcium foods: Eat foods totaling at least 1,200 mg of calcium every day.
Soy protein: Eat 20–25 grams of vegetable protein every day (in place of animal protein).
Total calorie intake: Eat your daily calorie intake goal.
Sodium: Eat no more than 1,500 mg of sodium every day.
Dark chocolate: Eat 2 tablespoons unsweetened dark cocoa powder (or 2 ounces dark chocolate) every day.
Red wine: Drink one to two 5-ounce glasses of red wine with food, every day.
Relaxation exercise: Perform some type of relaxation exercise such as deep breathing or meditation for at least 10 minutes every day.
Cardio exercise: Walk, swim, or bike for 30 minutes every day.

Notes:

Sample Day Illustrating the 10 Optimal BP-Lowering Lifestyle Strategies in Combination

Time/Meal	Food/Exercise	Minerals*				Calories†	Food	Other
		Na (mg)	K (mg)	Mg (mg)	Ca (mg)			
Early morning	45-minute walk, moderate intensity							cardio exercise
Breakfast	2/3 C old-fashioned oatmeal (dry)	4	196	74	28	204	Whole grains (2)	
	cooked with 1 C soy milk	124	287	61	61	131	Dairy subs. (1)	Soy protein (10 g)
	1 C cantaloupe balls	28	473	21	16	60	Fruit (1)	
	1 C orange juice	2	496	27	27	112	Fruit (1)	
	1 C coffee, black	5	116	7	5	2		
Snack	1 oz walnuts	1	123	44	27	183	Nuts (1)	
	1 oz dried apricots	3	325	9	15	67	Fruit (1)	
	1 6-oz cup light fat-free yogurt	85	250	27	240	100	Dairy (1)	
Lunch	Greek salad:							
	tomatoes, onions, cucumber, peppers, garlic	8	365	22	31	42	Vegetables (2)	
	2 green olives	76	1	0	1	8		
	0.6 oz low-fat feta cheese	235	–	–	50	35	Dairy (½)	
	dressed with							
	1 t olive oil, vinegar, and	0	0	0	0	40	Healthy oil (1)	
	fresh lemon juice							
	1 small whole-grain pita bread	340	109	44	10	74	Whole grains (2)	
	sandwich stuffed with:							
	1 Tb hummus +	36	26	4	7	27	Beans (½)	
	raw assorted vegetables	128	365	22	31	42	Vegetables (2)	
	1 C fat-free milk		410	27	504	86	Dairy (1)	

								Stress-management exercises
Early afternoon	10 minutes of progressive muscle relaxation and deep breathing exercises							
Snack	1 small apple	1	159	8	9	77	Fruit (1)	
	2 oz unsalted soy nuts	2	764	128	80	252	Beans (1)	Soy protein (24 g)
	6 cups air-popped popcorn	6	26	12	1	186	Whole grains (2)	
Dinner	1 glass red wine (5 oz)	6	187	18	18	125	Lean protein	Moderation of alcohol intake
	5-oz grilled salmon filet seasoned with garlic, dill, and fresh lemon juice	85	540	42	21	290		
	1 C brown rice	10	84	20	84	208	Whole grains (2)	
	2 C fresh spinach sautéed with garlic, 1 t olive oil, and fresh lemon juice	0	0	0	0	40	Vegetables (2) Healthy oil (1)	
	2 squares (2 oz) dark chocolate for dessert melted over 1 small banana (sliced)	3	100	32	11	84		Dark chocolate
		1	362	27	5	90	Fruit (1)	
	1 double decaffeinated espresso	8	70	48	1	0		
Daily Totals:		1,205	5,834	796	1,219	2,565		

*Recommended daily intakes: ≤ 1,500 mg sodium; ≥ 4,700 mg potassium; ≥ 500 mg magnesium; ≥ 1,200 mg calcium.

†The menu totals approximately 2,500 calories, designed for an individual requiring approximately 2,800 a day, thereby creating a daily calorie deficit (between diet and exercise) of about 500 calories a day. If followed for one week, this regimen would promote weight loss of approximately one pound.

Blood Pressure Down 4-Week Body Weight Graph

STARTING WEIGHT: _____ STARTING DATE: _____

Week 1 Weight _____	Week 2 Weight _____	Week 3 Weight _____	Week 4 Weight _____

Weight (lbs)

Starting weight   Week 1   Week 2   Week 3   Week 4

Appendix 3:

BODY MASS INDEX CALCULATIONS

Step 1: Your body weight in pounds: _____

Step 2: Your height in inches: _____

Step 3:
$$\text{BMI} = \left[\frac{\text{weight}}{(\text{height})^2}\right] \times 703$$

Step 4: Assess your number. A BMI of 18.5 to 25 is considered normal. A BMI over 25 is considered overweight and increases your risk of high blood pressure.

BMI calculation example:

Weight = 150 lbs
Height = 5'5" (65")
Calculation: $[150 \div (65)^2] \times 703 = 24.96$

Appendix 4:

BLOOD PRESSURE PROGRESS CHART

STARTING BP: _____ **STARTING DATE:** _____ **BLOOD PRESSURE DOWN WEEK:** 1 2 3 4

Monday	Tuesday	Wednesday	Thursday	Friday	Saturday	Sunday
AM reading #1:	AM reading #1:	AM reading #1:	AM reading #1:	AM reading #1:	AM reading #1:	AM reading #1:
AM reading #2:	AM reading #2:	AM reading #2:	AM reading #2:	AM reading #2:	AM reading #2:	AM reading #2:
AM reading #3:	AM reading #3:	AM reading #3:	AM reading #3:	AM reading #3:	AM reading #3:	AM reading #3:
Comments:	Comments:	Comments:	Comments:	Comments:	Comments:	Comments:
PM reading #1:	PM reading #1:	PM reading #1:	PM reading #1:	PM reading #1:	PM reading #1:	PM reading #1:
PM reading #2:	PM reading #2:	PM reading #2:	PM reading #2:	PM reading #2:	PM reading #2:	PM reading #2:
PM reading #3:	PM reading #3:	PM reading #3:	PM reading #3:	PM reading #3:	PM reading #3:	PM reading #3:
Comments:	Comments	Comments	Comments	Comments	Comments	Comments

Note: Blood pressure higher than 180/110 is a medical emergency. Call 911 immediately.
Remember: Take 2 to 3 blood pressure readings with at least 1 minute of rest in between measurements, and record all results.

Appendix 5:

CHEF CARD: SLASHING SALT AT RESTAURANTS

1. Copy and cut out this chef card, and keep it in your purse or wallet at all times.
2. Whenever you eat out, give this card to the chef or waiter for his or her help in verifying your meal will be healthful.
3. Remember, when eating out, watch portion sizes, as extra food equals extra sodium.

Cut along outline to cut out card

ATTENTION CHEF!

I am on a sodium-restricted diet for health purposes.
To help me avoid an elevation in my blood pressure, kindly avoid using any of the following "NO" ingredients in my food:

YES	NO
• Vinegars	• Any type of salt or sodium
• Citrus juices	• MSG
• Olive oil	• Broths and sauces (such as marinara and cheese sauces)
• Garlic, herbs, spices	• Asian condiments (such as soy sauces, teriyaki, miso)
• Wine (bottled, not cooking)	• Commercial dressings

thank you!

© *Blood Pressure Down: The 10-Step Plan to Lower Your Blood Pressure in 4 Weeks—Without Prescription Drugs* (Three Rivers Press; 2013).

Appendix 6:

MINERALS POCKET CHARTS

Cut along outlines to cut out cards

POTASSIUM	
Super-High*	**Very High****
Cantaloupe	Apricots
Casaba melon	Bananas
Honeydew melon	Dried fruits
Artichokes	Brussels sprouts
Avocado	Pumpkin
Beet greens	Cooked mushrooms
Cooked spinach	Chocolate (dark)
Swiss chard	Squash
White beans	Potatoes
Low-sodium V8	Kiwi
Prunes	

* Each food contains over 400 mg potassium per ½-cup serving
** Each food contains over 250 mg potassium per ½-cup serving

MAGNESIUM	
Super-High*	**Very High****
Cooked spinach	Brewed espresso
White beans	Clams
Corn	Brewed coffee
Swiss chard	Prickly pear cactus
Purslane	Peanut butter (low sodium)
Dry-roasted, unsalted	Avocado
almonds	Fat-free yogurt
Halibut	Kidney and pinto beans
Quinoa	Peas
Brown rice	Dry-roasted, unsalted peanuts
	Potato, baked, with skin

* Each food contains ~100 mg magnesium per typical serving
** Each food contains ~ 50 mg magnesium per typical serving

CALCIUM	
Super-High*	**Very High****
Nonfat plain yogurt	Tofu
Soy milk, fortified	
Fat-free milk	Canned salmon
Collard greens	
Cheeses:	Edamame
Low-sodium Parmesan, Swiss,	
mozzarella	Bok choy
Low-sodium and low-fat cottage	
cheese	Blackstrap molasses
Part-skim ricotta cheese	

* Each food contains over 300 mg calcium per typical serving
** Each food contains over 150 mg calcium per typical serving

Appendix 7:

SAMPLE BLOOD PRESSURE DOWN MEAL AND EXERCISE PLANS

Sample Week One: BLOOD PRESSURE DOWN MEAL AND EXERCISE PLANS

	Monday	Tuesday	Wednesday	Thursday	Friday	Saturday	Sunday
Exercise/ Supplements							
Breakfast	Buckwheat banana pancakes* Pumpkin oatmeal with yogurt and raisins*	Tofu scramble with avocado* Strawberry kiwi salad*	Oatmeal Cantaloupe yogurt parfaits* Chocolate soy milk	Chocolate smoothie with avocado and banana*	Puffed Wheat Soy milk Banana	Oatmeal Fresh blueberries Fresh banana	Puffed Wheat Soy milk Banana
Snack	Low-sodium V8 Raw almonds	Nonfat plain yogurt Pumpkin puree	Fresh orange Soy nuts	Soy nuts Fresh kiwi	Papaya banana salad*	Nonfat plain yogurt Pumpkin puree	Fresh orange
Lunch	Boca soy chicken patty Pepperidge Farm Whole Wheat Deli Flats White bean and broccoli salad* Mixed greens with balsamic Dijon vinaigrette*	Roasted almond butter* Pepperidge Farm Whole Wheat Deli Flats Banana Low-sodium V8	Tuna salad and spinach sandwiches* Garbanzo bean and spinach salad* Dark chocolate	Lentil soup with Swiss chard Mixed greens with balsamic Dijon vinaigrette* Whole-wheat roll Low-sodium V8	Eggless Tofu Salad* Mixed Greens with Balsamic Dijon vinaigrette* Pepperidge Farm Whole Wheat Deli Flats Fresh apple	Easy salmon cakes* Simple arugula salad* Strawberry kiwi salad*	Salmon black bean quesadillas* Fresh avocado dip* Warm edamame and corn salad*

	Monday	Tuesday	Wednesday	Thursday	Friday	Saturday	Sunday
Snack	Nonfat plain yogurt Pumpkin puree	Soy nut and apricot trail mix*	Fresh apple	Fresh banana Dark chocolate	Nonfat plain yogurt Pumpkin puree	Soy nuts	Tall soy latte
Dinner	Oven-roasted salmon with potatoes and tomatoes* Warm spinach and mushroom salad* Red wine	Meatless chili with portobello mushrooms* Baked potato with chive yogurt topping* Warm spinach and mushroom salad* Red wine	Dr. Janet's Easy roasted salmon* Garlic mashed potatoes* Spicy roasted broccoli* Red wine	Quick white clam sauce with whole-wheat spaghetti* Mixed greens with balsamic Dijon vinaigrette* Red wine	Slow-cooker turkey chili* Baked potato with chive yogurt topping* Mixed greens with balsamic Dijon vinaigrette* Red wine	Shrimp tacos with kiwi salsa* Black beans with sweet potato* Sautéed spinach with raisins and pistachios* Red wine	Penne pasta with lentils and kale* Red wine
Extras	Dark chocolate	European-style thick soy cocoa*	Nonfat plain yogurt Pumpkin puree	Nonfat plain yogurt Pumpkin puree sprinkled with cinnamon	Dark chocolate	Dark chocolate	Dark chocolate Nonfat plain yogurt Pumpkin puree Whipped topping

*Recipe provided in Appendix 8.

Sample Week Two: BLOOD PRESSURE DOWN MEAL AND EXERCISE PLANS

	Monday	Tuesday	Wednesday	Thursday	Friday	Saturday	Sunday
Exercise/ Supplements							
Breakfast	Buckwheat banana pancakes* Fresh cantaloupe	Puffed Wheat Soy milk Banana	Wheat bran toaster muffin Fresh banana Soy milk	Pumpkin oatmeal with yogurt and raisins* Soy milk	Chocolate smoothie with avocado and banana*	Tofu scramble with avocado* Cantaloupe yogurt parfaits*	Pumpkin oatmeal with yogurt and raisins* Fresh banana Soy milk
Snack	Nonfat plain yogurt Pumpkin puree	Nonfat plain yogurt Pumpkin puree	Papaya banana salad*	Raw almonds	Fruit salad with poppy seed yogurt dressing*	Nonfat plain yogurt Pumpkin puree	Stawberry kiwi salad*
Lunch	Falafel patty Whole-wheat pita Tomato Spinach Cucumber slices Tzatziki sauce Low-sodium V8 Fresh banana	Roasted vegetables with quinoa and spinach* Lentil soup with Swiss chard* Mixed greens with balsamic Dijon vinaigrette*	Simple arugula salad* Lentil and tempeh stew* Fresh apple	Eggless tofu salad* Pepperidge Farm Whole Wheat Deli Flats Garbanzo bean and spinach salad*	Tuna salad and spinach sandwiches* Soy nut and apricot trail mix* Fresh apple	Roasted almond butter* Pepperidge Farm Whole Wheat Deli Flats Fresh banana Soy milk	Boca soy chicken patty White bean and broccoli salad* Low-sodium V8

	Monday	Tuesday	Wednesday	Thursday	Friday	Saturday	Sunday
Snack	Soy nut and apricot trail mix*	Low-sodium V8	European-style thick soy cocoa*	Nonfat plain yogurt	Nonfat plain yogurt	Soy crisps	Nonfat plain yogurt
	Soy milk			Pumpkin puree	Pumpkin puree	Fresh apple	Pumpkin puree
Dinner	Dr. Janet's Roasted tofu and cauliflower curry with brown rice*	Slow-cooker turkey chili*	Dr. Janet's Easy roasted salmon*	Salmon black bean quesadillas*	Creamy Cannellini bean with spinach soup*	Easy roasted salmon*	Shrimp tacos with kiwi salsa*
	Mixed greens with balsamic Dijon vinaigrette*	Baked potato with chive yogurt topping*	Spicy roasted broccoli*	Fresh avocado dip*	Boca Soy Chicken Patty	Roasted sweet potato fries*	Apricot and almond buckwheat pilaf*
	Red wine	Red wine	Red wine	Black beans with sweet potato*	Pepperidge Farm Whole Wheat Deli Flats	Spicy roasted broccoli*	Mixed greens with balsamic Dijon vinaigrette*
				Apricot and almond buckwheat pilaf*	Warm herbed potato salad*	Warm spinach and mushroom salad*	Red wine
				Red wine	Red wine		
Extras	Dark cholcolate	Dark chocolate	Nonfat plain yogurt	Papaya banana salad*	2 almond thumbprint cookies*	Janet's Chocolate banana cake*	Dark chocolate
			Pumpkin puree	Dark chocolate		Red wine	
			Whipped topping				

*Recipe provided in Appendix 8.

Appendix 8:

HEART-HEALTHY RECIPES

Note: computerized nutrition analyses were performed using arbitrary recipe serving sizes (portions that I typically eat) and not using standardized "serving sizes" listed under the USDA guidelines. In all the following recipes, whenever possible, I recommend using organically grown fruits, vegetables, grains, and other products; fish that has been caught in the wild; and free-range poultry that has been raised without hormones and antibiotics.

Notes about using the Blood Pressure Down recipes:

- Cooking without salt is a liberating experience! In our recipes we eliminated salt and added a host of other fresh ingredients to boost flavors.
- Make cooking without salt a delicious endeavor. For success with these recipes, keep on hand ingredients such as fresh lemons, fresh herbs such as cilantro, parsley, and basil, fresh garlic cloves, flavorful olive oil, red wine vinegar, and spices such as cumin, curry powder, and crushed red pepper flakes.
- In our recipes we take advantage of cooking methods, such as roasting and sautéing, that caramelize and bring out the natural sweetness in vegetables. Don't skip this important step even when starting a soup or stew.

- In place of salt, we used Mrs. Dash Original salt-free seasoning blend. It provides a nice balance of flavor without any of the bitter overtones that can be prominent in No-Salt or other potassium chloride salt substitutes.
- When starting to cook without salt, give your taste buds several weeks to acclimate to not having salt in your food. Even though the recipes are full of flavor, your tongue will miss the salt at first. Be patient as you start to enjoy other flavors in food. The wait is worth it for your blood pressure and your health!
- The ingredients in these recipes are readily available at large supermarkets. Buy fresh produce in season when possible, and organic vegetables if affordable.

Week One

Monday's Recipes

BUCKWHEAT BANANA PANCAKES

YIELD: EIGHT 4-INCH PANCAKES

SERVES 8

Buckwheat flour adds a hearty flavor to these pancakes with a ripe banana mixed into the batter.

- ¼ cup all-purpose flour
- ¼ cup buckwheat flour
- ½ teaspoon baking soda
- ½ teaspoon baking powder
- ½ cup mashed banana (about 1 medium banana)
- ½ cup buttermilk
- 1 large egg
- 1 tablespoon canola oil
- 1 tablespoon molasses

In a bowl whisk together the all-purpose flour, buckwheat flour, baking soda, and baking powder. In another bowl mash the banana with the buttermilk, egg, oil, and molasses. Fold in the flour mixture and mix just until blended. Spray a griddle with nonstick cooking spray and heat. Using a ¼-cup measuring cup, ladle the batter onto the hot griddle. Cook the pancakes until the edges appear dry and bubbles are breaking through the surface of the pancakes. Flip the cakes and cook on the other side until golden brown. Keep warm in a 200°F oven.

NUTRITION PER PANCAKE

CALORIES	SODIUM	POTASSIUM	MAGNESIUM	CALCIUM	FAT*
78 kcal	128 mg	144 mg	23 mg	50 mg	3 g

SATURATED FAT	CHOLESTEROL	CARBOHYDRATE	DIETARY FIBER	SUGARS	PROTEIN
<1 g	27 mg	12 g	<1 g	4 g	2 g

* FAT: EPA 0 g, DHA 0 g, ALA 0 g

PUMPKIN OATMEAL WITH YOGURT AND RAISINS

SERVES 4

A warm bowl of oatmeal filled with spices and pumpkin is a cold-weather crowd pleaser. This is so easy to make in the microwave.

1½ cups water
½ teaspoon ground cinnamon
1 cup old-fashioned oats
½ cup canned pumpkin puree
¼ cup raisins
1 tablespoon molasses
½ cup sugar-free vanilla yogurt, divided
4 tablespoons chopped walnuts, divided

In an 8-cup microwave-safe dish stir together the water, cinnamon, and oats. Place in the microwave and cook on high power for 4 to 5 minutes or until most of the liquid is absorbed. Remove from the microwave and stir in the pumpkin puree, raisins, and molasses. Spoon into 4 bowls and top each with 2 tablespoons yogurt and 1 tablespoon chopped walnuts. Serve immediately.

NUTRITION PER SERVING

CALORIES	SODIUM	POTASSIUM	MAGNESIUM	CALCIUM	FAT*
188 kcal	23 mg	410 mg	66 mg	117 mg	6 g

SATURATED FAT	CHOLESTEROL	CARBOHYDRATE	DIETARY FIBER	SUGARS	PROTEIN
<1 g	1 mg	30 g	4 g	12 g	6 g

* FAT: EPA 0 g, DHA 0 g, ALA 0 g

WHITE BEAN AND BROCCOLI SALAD

YIELD: 4 CUPS

SERVES 8

Rich and creamy, with cannellini beans and a fresh yogurt dressing.

> One 15-ounce can cannellini beans, drained and rinsed
> (about 1½ cups)
> 2 cups chopped fresh broccoli (about ½ small head)
> 2 scallions, thinly sliced
> ½ red bell pepper, seeded and chopped (about ½ cup)
> ¼ cup chopped fresh basil
> ¼ cup low-fat plain yogurt
> 2 tablespoons red wine vinegar
> 2 tablespoons olive oil
> ½ teaspoon salt-free seasoning blend
> ½ teaspoon freshly ground black pepper

In a salad bowl mix the cannellini beans, broccoli, scallions, red pepper, and basil. Whisk together in a small bowl the yogurt, vinegar, olive oil, salt-free seasoning blend, and pepper. Pour over the salad ingredients and mix gently.

NUTRITION PER ½-CUP SERVING

CALORIES	SODIUM	POTASSIUM	MAGNESIUM	CALCIUM	FAT*
92 kcal	14 mg	391 mg	30 mg	60 mg	4 g

SATURATED FAT	CHOLESTEROL	CARBOHYDRATE	DIETARY FIBER	SUGARS	PROTEIN
<1 g	1 mg	11 g	<3 g	1 g	4 g

* FAT: EPA 0 g, DHA 0 g, ALA 0 g

MIXED GREENS WITH BALSAMIC DIJON VINAIGRETTE

YIELD: 8 CUPS SALAD

SERVES 4

4 cups mixed salad greens

4 cups fresh baby spinach

¼ cup roasted pumpkin seed kernels

¼ cup diced dried apricots

½ cup balsamic Dijon vinaigrette (recipe below)

In a shallow salad bowl, toss the salad greens and baby spinach with ¼ cup of the dressing. Sprinkle with pumpkin seeds and apricots. Drizzle with ¼ cup more of the remaining dressing. Serve immediately.

NUTRITION PER 2 CUPS SALAD AND 2 TABLESPOONS DRESSING

CALORIES	SODIUM	POTASSIUM	MAGNESIUM	CALCIUM	FAT*
116 kcal	36 mg	530 mg	110 mg	62 mg	8 g

SATURATED FAT	CHOLESTEROL	CARBOHYDRATE	DIETARY FIBER	SUGARS	PROTEIN
3 g	0 mg	10 g	2 g	4 g	6 g

* FAT: EPA 0 g, DHA 0 g, ALA 0 g

DR. JANET'S BALSAMIC DIJON VINAIGRETTE

YIELD: 6 OUNCES (¾ CUP)

SERVES 12

Homemade salad dressings and vinaigrettes are easy to make, and lower in sodium than most prepared dressings.

2 tablespoons minced shallots
2 tablespoons Dijon mustard
¼ cup balsamic vinegar
¼ cup purple grape juice
¼ teaspoon dried basil
½ teaspoon dried oregano
1 tablespoon molasses
¼ cup extra virgin olive oil

Combine the shallots, mustard, vinegar, grape juice, basil, oregano, molasses, and olive oil in a blender and blend until well mixed.

NUTRITION PER 1-TABLESPOON SERVING

CALORIES	SODIUM	POTASSIUM	MAGNESIUM	CALCIUM	FAT*
51 kcal	34 mg	63 mg	6 mg	20 mg	4 g

SATURATED FAT	CHOLESTEROL	CARBOHYDRATE	DIETARY FIBER	SUGARS	PROTEIN
1 g	0 mg	3 g	<1 g	1 g	<1 g

* FAT: EPA 0 g, DHA 0 g, ALA 0 g

OVEN-ROASTED SALMON
WITH POTATOES AND TOMATOES

SERVES 4

Fresh fish and vegetables, roasted in a hot oven, makes a quick and delicious meal with very little preparation. Cod can be substituted for the salmon if desired.

> Four 6-ounce salmon fillets
> 3 tablespoons olive oil, divided
> 1 teaspoon salt-free seasoning blend
> ½ teaspoon freshly ground black pepper
> 2 pounds small red potatoes, washed and quartered
> 4 cloves garlic, peeled and halved
> ½ teaspoon dried rosemary
> ½ teaspoon dried thyme
> 2 cups grape tomatoes, halved
> Juice of one lemon
> ¼ cup minced parsley

Preheat oven to 450°F. Drizzle the salmon with 1 tablespoon olive oil and sprinkle with salt-free seasoning blend and pepper. Refrigerate until ready to use.

On a rimmed baking sheet toss potatoes with garlic, rosemary, thyme, salt-free seasoning blend, pepper, and the remaining 2 tablespoons olive oil. Turn as many cut-sides of the potatoes down as possible. Bake for about 20 minutes, just until the potatoes start to brown. Remove baking sheet from the oven and add the tomatoes to the potatoes, stirring to combine. Push the potatoes to one side and lay the prepared salmon on the pan next to the vegetables. Return to the oven and bake until the fish is cooked through and the potatoes are brown and tender, about 20 minutes. Remove from the oven and squeeze lemon juice over the top and sprinkle with fresh chopped parsley.

NUTRITION PER 1 PIECE SALMON AND ONE-QUARTER OF VEGETABLES

CALORIES	SODIUM	POTASSIUM	MAGNESIUM	CALCIUM	FAT*
519 kcal	98 mg	2,080 mg	111 mg	63 mg	22 g

SATURATED FAT	CHOLESTEROL	CARBOHYDRATE	DIETARY FIBER	SUGARS	PROTEIN
3 g	94 mg	41 g	5 g	3 g	39 g

* FAT: EPA 1 g, DHA 2 g, ALA 0 g

WARM SPINACH AND MUSHROOM SALAD

YIELD: 8 CUPS SALAD AND ½ CUP DRESSING

SERVES 4

The dressing can be made ahead of time and refrigerated. (Just warm it up in the microwave for 30 seconds before serving, using care not to boil it.)

¼ cup olive oil
¼ cup diced yellow onion
¼ cup water
2 tablespoons red wine vinegar
2 tablespoons molasses
2 tablespoons Dijon mustard
½ teaspoon sweet paprika
Dash liquid smoke
½ teaspoon freshly ground black pepper
4 cups fresh baby spinach (about 5 ounces)
One 8-ounce box sliced white mushrooms
1 cup grape or cherry tomatoes, cut into quarters

In a small skillet heat olive oil over medium-low heat. Add the onions and cook until softened and golden, about 5 minutes. In a blender combine the cooked onions and the oil, water, vinegar, molasses, Dijon, paprika, liquid smoke, and pepper. Pulse on high speed until smooth.

Place the spinach in a large salad bowl. Cut the mushroom slices in half and place on top of the spinach. Toss the spinach and mushrooms with the warm dressing and garnish with tomatoes.

NUTRITION PER 2 CUPS SALAD PLUS 2 TABLESPOONS DRESSING

CALORIES	SODIUM	POTASSIUM	MAGNESIUM	CALCIUM	FAT*
179 kcal	178 mg	539 mg	49 mg	62 mg	15 g

SATURATED FAT	CHOLESTEROL	CARBOHYDRATE	DIETARY FIBER	SUGARS	PROTEIN
2 g	0 mg	11 g	2 g	4 g	4 g

* FAT: EPA 0 g, DHA 0 g, ALA 0 g

Tuesday's Recipes

TOFU SCRAMBLE WITH AVOCADO
SERVES 2

Packed with soy protein and spices, this scramble is an easy and nourishing way to start any day. If desired, fresh salsa can be substituted for the avocado and the tomatoes.

> **2 tablespoons olive oil**
> **7 ounces soft tofu (not silken) (half of one 14-ounce package)**
> **½ teaspoon ground turmeric**
> **½ teaspoon salt-free seasoning blend**
> **¼ teaspoon freshly ground black pepper**
> **½ cup egg substitute**
> **½ avocado, pitted, peeled, and cubed**
> **½ cup grape tomatoes, quartered**

In a large nonstick skillet, heat oil over medium-high heat. Pat the tofu dry with a paper towel. Crumble tofu into the skillet. Sprinkle with turmeric and season with salt-free seasoning blend and pepper. Cook, stirring gently, until most of the moisture is cooked out of the tofu, about 4 minutes. Meanwhile, in a bowl whisk together the egg substitute, salt substitute, and pepper. Set aside.

When the tofu appears dry, reduce the heat to medium. Pour the reserved eggs over the tofu. Cook, stirring occasionally for about 2 minutes until set. Divide between two plates and serve topped with chopped avocado and tomatoes.

NUTRITION PER SERVING

CALORIES	SODIUM	POTASSIUM	MAGNESIUM	CALCIUM	FAT*
208 kcal	95 mg	523 mg	45 mg	120 mg	15 g

SATURATED FAT	CHOLESTEROL	CARBOHYDRATE	DIETARY FIBER	SUGARS	PROTEIN
2 g	0 mg	9 g	4 g	1 g	13 g

* FAT: EPA 0 g, DHA 0 g, ALA 0.1 g

STRAWBERRY KIWI SALAD

YIELD: 5 CUPS

SERVES 5

The ripeness of strawberries and kiwi varies seasonally. If you like, sweeten to taste with 1 tablespoon honey or Splenda.

1 pound strawberries, hulled and sliced
2 kiwis, peeled and diced
1 medium cucumber, peeled, seeded, and diced
1 jalapeño, seeded and minced
2 tablespoons chopped fresh mint leaves
Juice of half a lemon (about 1 tablespoon)

Place strawberries, kiwis, cucumber, jalapeño, mint, and 1 tablespoon lemon juice in a medium bowl and toss until combined. Set aside.

NUTRITION PER 1-CUP SERVING

CALORIES	SODIUM	POTASSIUM	MAGNESIUM	CALCIUM	FAT*
57 kcal	3 mg	316 mg	24 mg	36 mg	1 g

SATURATED FAT	CHOLESTEROL	CARBOHYDRATE	DIETARY FIBER	SUGARS	PROTEIN
<1 g	0 mg	14 g	3 g	7 g	1 g

* FAT: EPA 0 g, DHA 0 g, ALA 0 g

ROASTED ALMOND BUTTER

YIELD: ⅔ CUP

SERVES 10

Simple and inexpensive to prepare at home, and a good source of calcium, magnesium, and healthy fats. All you need is a little patience and a good food processor! Be sure not to use roasted or salted almonds.

6 ounces whole unsalted almonds

Preheat the oven to 350°F. Place the almonds on a baking sheet. Bake for about 15 minutes, until fragrant, stirring once or twice to prevent burning. Pour almonds off the baking sheet onto a heatproof plate or a piece of aluminum foil to cool to room temperature. Pour the cooled almonds into a food processor and turn on the processor. Let the processor run for about 2 minutes and then scrape down the sides of the processor. The nuts will appear loosely chopped. Continue to process until the almonds form clumps; the clumps will then turn into a ball, then finally loosen up and turn more smooth as it starts to look more and more like almond butter. Scrape down the sides. This will take a total of about 4 to 5 minutes of processing.

NUTRITION PER 2-TABLESPOON SERVING

CALORIES	SODIUM	POTASSIUM	MAGNESIUM	CALCIUM	FAT*
100 kcal	2 mg	132 mg	52 mg	48 mg	9 g

SATURATED FAT	CHOLESTEROL	CARBOHYDRATE	DIETARY FIBER	SUGARS	PROTEIN
1 g	0 mg	4 g	2 g	0 g	4 g

* FAT: EPA 0 g, DHA 0 g, ALA 0 g

SOY NUT AND APRICOT TRAIL MIX

YIELD: 5 CUPS

This nutty, potassium-rich snack is quick to mix.

- 1 cup roasted soy nuts
- 1 cup roasted shelled pistachios
- 1 cup pumpkin seeds
- 1 cup dried apricots, chopped
- 1 cup raisins

Mix all ingredients in a bowl. Scoop into ¼-cup portions and place each portion in a zip-top snack bag.

NUTRITION PER ¼-CUP SERVING

CALORIES	SODIUM	POTASSIUM	MAGNESIUM	CALCIUM	FAT*
198 kcal	4 mg	487 mg	106 mg	40 mg	11 g

SATURATED FAT	CHOLESTEROL	CARBOHYDRATE	DIETARY FIBER	SUGARS	PROTEIN
2 g	0 mg	18 g	3 g	8 g	11 g

* FAT: EPA 0 g, DHA 0 g, ALA 0 g

MEATLESS CHILI WITH PORTOBELLO MUSHROOMS

YIELD: 10 CUPS

SERVES 8

Meaty portobello mushroom caps make this chili hearty and filling. Wipe the mushrooms with a damp paper towel and pull off the stems before using.

        2 tablespoons olive oil
        1 large onion, peeled and diced
        1 large red bell pepper, seeded and chopped
        1 large green bell pepper, seeded and chopped
        1 jalapeño pepper, seeded and chopped
        2 cups peeled and chopped carrots
        4 portobello mushroom caps (about 1 pound), stems removed, cut into
            chunks
        2 cloves garlic, peeled and minced
        2 tablespoons chili powder
        1 tablespoon ground cumin
        1 tablespoon salt-free seasoning blend
        4 cups low-sodium vegetable juice
        One 10-ounce can diced tomatoes with green chilies, drained
        1 cup frozen corn kernels
        One 15-ounce can black beans, drained and rinsed (about 1½ cups)
        One 15-ounce can kidney beans, drained and rinsed (about 1½ cups)
        1 cup water
        1 teaspoon Worcestershire sauce

In a large pot heat the olive oil over medium heat. Add the onion, bell peppers, jalapeño pepper, and carrots. Stir and cook for 5 minutes to soften. Add the mushrooms, garlic, chili powder, ground cumin, and salt-free seasoning blend. Stir to coat the mushroom chunks with the spices and cook for about 3 minutes until the mushrooms start to sweat and release some of their juice. Stir in the vegetable juice, diced tomatoes, corn, beans, water, and Worcestershire sauce. Simmer over low heat for about 1 hour until thick and the vegetables are tender.

NUTRITION PER 1¼-CUP SERVING

CALORIES	SODIUM	POTASSIUM	MAGNESIUM	CALCIUM	FAT*
219 kcal	283 mg	1,103 mg	81 mg	76 mg	5 g

SATURATED FAT	CHOLESTEROL	CARBOHYDRATE	DIETARY FIBER	SUGARS	PROTEIN
1 g	0 mg	38 g	10 g	6 g	6 g

* FAT: EPA 0 g, DHA 0 g, ALA 0 g

BAKED POTATO WITH CHIVE YOGURT TOPPING

YIELD: 4 POTATOES

SERVES 4

Easy-to-bake potatoes are topped with a delicious herb-enhanced sauce.

> Four 8-ounce baking potatoes
> ½ cup plain nonfat yogurt
> 1 tablespoon olive oil
> 2 tablespoons chopped chives
> Zest of one lemon
> 1 teaspoon salt-free seasoning blend
> ¼ teaspoon freshly ground black pepper

Preheat oven to 400°F. Poke the surface of the potatoes several times with a fork; then place them on a baking sheet. Bake for about 1 hour to 1 hour and 10 minutes or until easily pierced with a fork. Meanwhile, in a separate bowl, whisk together the yogurt, olive oil, chives, lemon zest, salt-free seasoning, and pepper. Just before serving use a knife to cut a slit in the top of each potato. Pull the potatoes open to expose the cooked flesh and spoon 2 tablespoons of yogurt topping onto each potato.

NUTRITION PER 1 POTATO WITH 2 TABLESPOONS YOGURT TOPPING

CALORIES	SODIUM	POTASSIUM	MAGNESIUM	CALCIUM	FAT*
218 kcal	32 mg	966 mg	55 mg	86 mg	4 g

SATURATED FAT	CHOLESTEROL	CARBOHYDRATE	DIETARY FIBER	SUGARS	PROTEIN
<1 g	2 mg	41 g	3 g	4 g	6 g

* FAT: EPA 0 g, DHA 0 g, ALA 0 g

DR. JANET'S EUROPEAN-STYLE THICK SOY COCOA

YIELD: 2 CUPS

SERVES 4

Thick and rich, this soy cocoa is good morning, noon, or night.

- ½ cup unsweetened cocoa powder
- 2 tablespoons Splenda Brown Sugar Blend
- 1 tablespoon cornstarch
- ⅛ teaspoon ground cinnamon
- 2 cups vanilla soy milk

In a saucepan mix cocoa, sugar, cornstarch, and cinnamon. Whisk in 1 cup soy milk to make a thick paste and to dissolve the dry ingredients. This will look like thick chocolate frosting. Whisk in the remaining 1 cup soy milk until smooth. Place over low heat and stir until steaming and thick. Do not boil. Serve hot.

NUTRITION PER ½-CUP SERVING

CALORIES	SODIUM	POTASSIUM	MAGNESIUM	CALCIUM	FAT*
137 kcal	71 mg	330 mg	85 mg	37 mg	4 g

SATURATED FAT	CHOLESTEROL	CARBOHYDRATE	DIETARY FIBER	SUGARS	PROTEIN
1 g	0 mg	24 g	5 g	6 g	8 g

* FAT: EPA 0 g, DHA 0 g, ALA 0 g

Wednesday's Recipes

CANTALOUPE YOGURT PARFAITS

SERVES 4

This is also delicious with other high-potassium fruits such as bananas, fresh apricots, honeydew melon, or kiwi layered with, or in place of, the cantaloupe.

> 2 cups diced cantaloupe (from about ½ medium-sized cantaloupe)
> 1 cup vanilla low-fat yogurt
> ¼ cup chopped pistachios

Layer the diced cantaloupe and yogurt in parfait or wine glasses. Garnish with chopped pistachios.

NUTRITION PER SERVING

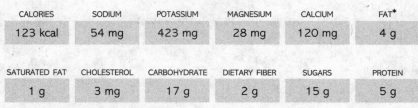

CALORIES	SODIUM	POTASSIUM	MAGNESIUM	CALCIUM	FAT*
123 kcal	54 mg	423 mg	28 mg	120 mg	4 g

SATURATED FAT	CHOLESTEROL	CARBOHYDRATE	DIETARY FIBER	SUGARS	PROTEIN
1 g	3 mg	17 g	2 g	15 g	5 g

* FAT: EPA 0 g, DHA 0 g, ALA 0 g

TUNA SALAD AND SPINACH SANDWICHES

YIELD: 2 CUPS TUNA

SERVES 4

One 6.4-ounce pouch light tuna packed in water

½ medium cucumber, peeled, seeded, and diced

½ small red onion, peeled and diced (about ¼ cup)

2 ribs celery, diced

½ teaspoon dill weed

2 tablespoons olive oil

Juice of one lemon

½ teaspoon salt-free seasoning blend

¼ teaspoon freshly ground black pepper

8 slices 100 percent whole-wheat sandwich bread

1 cup fresh baby spinach

Flake the tuna with a fork in a bowl. Add the cucumber, onion, celery, and dill weed. Drizzle with the olive oil and lemon juice and stir to combine. Season with salt-free seasoning blend and pepper. Lay 4 slices of bread on a clean countertop. Top each with ½ cup tuna salad and ¼ cup baby spinach leaves. Top with another slice of bread and press down to compact the tuna and the spinach. Serve immediately.

NUTRITION PER SANDWICH (½ CUP TUNA)

CALORIES	SODIUM	POTASSIUM	MAGNESIUM	CALCIUM	FAT*
194 kcal	450 mg	410 mg	79 mg	81 mg	3 g

SATURATED FAT	CHOLESTEROL	CARBOHYDRATE	DIETARY FIBER	SUGARS	PROTEIN
<1 g	14 g	27 g	4 g	1 g	17 g

* FAT: EPA <1 g, DHA <1 g, ALA 0 g

GARBANZO BEAN AND SPINACH SALAD

YIELD: 5 CUPS

SERVES 10

Heart-healthy spinach is chopped and mixed with garbanzo beans for a refreshing bean salad.

Two 15-ounce cans garbanzo beans, drained and rinsed (3 cups cooked)
½ small red onion, peeled and finely chopped (about ¼ cup)
4 cups fresh baby spinach leaves (about 5 ounces)
3 tablespoons olive oil
1 tablespoon Dijon mustard
1 teaspoon dried basil
Juice of half a lemon (about 1 tablespoon)
1 teaspoon salt-free seasoning blend
½ teaspoon freshly ground black pepper

In large bowl mix the beans and onion. Chop the spinach into small pieces and add to the beans. In a small bowl whisk together the oil, mustard, basil, lemon juice, salt-free seasoning blend, and pepper. Mix into bean mixture to combine. Serve immediately or store refrigerated until ready to serve.

NUTRITION PER ½-CUP SERVING

CALORIES	SODIUM	POTASSIUM	MAGNESIUM	CALCIUM	FAT*
132 kcal	30 mg	232 mg	32 mg	41 mg	6 g

SATURATED FAT	CHOLESTEROL	CARBOHYDRATE	DIETARY FIBER	SUGARS	PROTEIN
<1 g	0 mg	16 g	4 g	<1 g	5 g

* FAT: EPA 0 g, DHA 0 g, ALA 0 g

DR. JANET'S EASY ROASTED SALMON

SERVES 4

Four 6-ounce wild salmon fillets
One lemon, cut into 4 wedges
Freshly ground black pepper
¼ cup minced fresh dill (from one small bunch)
4 cloves garlic, peeled and minced

Preheat oven to 400°F. Spray a 13-by-9-by-2-inch glass baking dish with nonstick spray. Place the salmon fillets in the baking dish. Squeeze juice from one wedge of lemon over each fillet. Sprinkle the salmon with black pepper, chopped fresh dill, and minced garlic. Bake until salmon is opaque in the center, about 20 to 22 minutes.

NUTRITION PER 6-OUNCE SERVING

CALORIES	SODIUM	POTASSIUM	MAGNESIUM	CALCIUM	FAT*
251 kcal	78 mg	894 mg	53 mg	36 mg	11 g

SATURATED FAT	CHOLESTEROL	CARBOHYDRATE	DIETARY FIBER	SUGARS	PROTEIN
2 g	94 mg	2 g	<1 g	<1 g	34 g

* FAT: EPA 1 g, DHA 2 g, ALA 0 g

SPICY ROASTED BROCCOLI

YIELD: 8 CUPS

SERVES 8

1¼ pounds broccoli, large stems trimmed and cut into 2-inch pieces
   (about 8 cups)
4 tablespoons olive oil, divided
½ teaspoon salt-free seasoning blend
¼ teaspoon freshly ground black pepper
4 cloves garlic, peeled and minced
¼ teaspoon crushed red pepper flakes

Preheat the oven to 450°F. In a large bowl toss together the broccoli and 2 table-spoons olive oil. Sprinkle with salt-free seasoning blend and pepper. Transfer to a rimmed baking sheet and bake for 15 minutes. Meanwhile mix together 2 table-spoons oil, garlic, and red pepper flakes. After the broccoli has cooked 15 minutes, drizzle the garlic oil over the broccoli and shake the baking sheet to coat the broccoli. Return to the oven and continue baking until the broccoli starts to brown, about 8 to 10 more minutes. Serve hot.

NUTRITION PER 1-CUP SERVING

CALORIES	SODIUM	POTASSIUM	MAGNESIUM	CALCIUM	FAT*
86 kcal	24 mg	232 mg	16 mg	37 mg	7 g

SATURATED FAT	CHOLESTEROL	CARBOHYDRATE	DIETARY FIBER	SUGARS	PROTEIN
1 g	0 mg	5 g	2 g	1 g	2 g

* FAT: EPA 0 g, DHA 0 g, ALA 0 g

GARLIC MASHED POTATOES

YIELD: 8 CUPS

SERVES 8

A creamy alternative to traditional mashed potatoes.

> 2 pounds all-purpose red or Yukon gold potatoes, scrubbed and cut
> into large chunks
> 6 cloves garlic, peeled
> ¼ cup olive oil
> 1 teaspoon salt-free seasoning blend
> ½ teaspoon freshly ground black pepper

In a large saucepan place the potato chunks and peeled garlic cloves. Cover with cold water and bring to a boil. Reduce the heat and cook for about 25 minutes or until the potatoes are tender when pierced with a fork. Remove from heat. Measure out and reserve ¾ cup of the cooking liquid. Drain the rest of the cooking liquid off the potatoes. Add the olive oil, salt-free seasoning blend, pepper, and reserved cooking liquid to the potatoes. Mash with a handheld potato masher or large fork. Taste and season with more salt and pepper if desired.

NUTRITION PER 1-CUP SERVING

CALORIES	SODIUM	POTASSIUM	MAGNESIUM	CALCIUM	FAT*
145 kcal	7 mg	527 mg	26 mg	16 mg	7 g

SATURATED FAT	CHOLESTEROL	CARBOHYDRATE	DIETARY FIBER	SUGARS	PROTEIN
1 g	0 mg	19 g	2 g	1 g	2 g

* FAT: EPA 0 g, DHA 0 g, ALA 0 g

Thursday's Recipes

CHOCOLATE SMOOTHIE WITH AVOCADO AND BANANA

SERVES 2

A rich smoothie that harnesses the antioxidant power of unsweetened cocoa powder.

> 2 cups vanilla soy milk
> ½ avocado, pitted and peeled
> One medium banana, peeled
> ¼ cup unsweetened cocoa powder
> 2 individual packets Splenda

Place all ingredients in a blender and process until smooth. Serve immediately.

NUTRITION PER 12-OUNCE SERVING

CALORIES	SODIUM	POTASSIUM	MAGNESIUM	CALCIUM	FAT*
252 kcal	102 mg	822 mg	122 mg	390 mg	12 g

SATURATED FAT	CHOLESTEROL	CARBOHYDRATE	DIETARY FIBER	SUGARS	PROTEIN
2 g	0 mg	33 g	8 g	8 g	11 g

* FAT: EPA 0 g, DHA 0 g, ALA <1 g

LENTIL SOUP WITH SWISS CHARD

SERVES 12

Extra portions can be easily frozen, then thawed and reheated when a quick meal is in order.

  2 tablespoons olive oil
  1 large onion, peeled and chopped
  4 carrots, peeled and finely chopped
  1½ teaspoons dried thyme
  1 teaspoon dried oregano or basil
  One 28-ounce can low-salt diced tomatoes, with their juice
  One 6-ounce can low-salt tomato paste
  8 cups reduced-sodium chicken or vegetable broth
  4 cups water
  2½ cups lentils (about 1 pound), rinsed and picked over
  1 teaspoon salt-free seasoning blend
  ½ teaspoon freshly ground black pepper
  ¾ cup dry red wine
  2 cups chopped Swiss chard

In a Dutch oven heat oil over medium heat. Add onion, carrot, thyme, and oregano and cook for 10 minutes until softened. Add the tomatoes (and their juice), tomato paste, broth, water, and lentils. Bring the soup to a boil, reduce the heat, cover the pan and simmer the soup for about 1 hour or until the lentils are tender. Stir in the salt-free seasoning blend, pepper, wine, and chard and simmer for 15 more minutes until the chard is cooked.

NUTRITION PER SERVING

CALORIES	SODIUM	POTASSIUM	MAGNESIUM	CALCIUM	FAT*
213 kcal	245 mg	875 mg	67 mg	69 mg	3 g

SATURATED FAT	CHOLESTEROL	CARBOHYDRATE	DIETARY FIBER	SUGARS	PROTEIN
<1 g	0 mg	32 g	15 g	5 g	15 g

* FAT: EPA 0 g, DHA 0 g, ALA 0 g

QUICK WHITE CLAM SAUCE
WITH WHOLE-WHEAT SPAGHETTI

YIELD: 2 CUPS SAUCE AND 4 CUPS COOKED SPAGHETTI

SERVES 4

Serve this quick sauce over long, thin pasta such as whole-wheat spaghetti or linguine.

        8 ounces uncooked whole-wheat spaghetti

        4 tablespoons olive oil, divided

        ½ medium yellow onion, peeled and chopped

        4 carrots, peeled, and shredded or chopped fine

        4 cloves garlic, peeled and minced

        ½ teaspoon crushed red pepper flakes

        ¼ cup dry white wine

        1 cup low-sodium chicken broth

        ½ cup chopped fresh parsley

        Two 6-ounce cans chopped clams, drained and rinsed

        ½ teaspoon salt-free seasoning blend

        ¼ teaspoon freshly ground black pepper

Bring a large pot of water to a boil. Add the pasta and cook for 7 to 8 minutes, or until desired degree of doneness. Drain well and rinse with hot water if desired to keep pasta from sticking together. Keep warm until sauce is ready.

Meanwhile, in a large skillet over medium heat, heat 2 tablespoons olive oil. Add the onion and carrot. Cook stirring until soft, about 4 minutes. Stir in the garlic and red pepper flakes. Cook for 1 more minute until the garlic is fragrant. Stir in the white wine, increase the heat to medium high, and cook until the wine is reduced and slightly thickened, about 2 minutes. Slowly whisk in the remaining 2 tablespoons olive oil and the chicken broth. Bring to a boil and cook for about 2 more minutes to thicken. Stir in the chopped parsley and clams. Heat through about 1 minute; season with salt-free seasoning blend and fresh black pepper.

Serve immediately over hot pasta.

NUTRITION PER 1/2 CUP SAUCE AND 1 CUP PASTA SERVING

CALORIES	SODIUM	POTASSIUM	MAGNESIUM	CALCIUM	FAT*
497 kcal	220 mg	994 mg	113 mg	147 mg	16 g

SATURATED FAT	CHOLESTEROL	CARBOHYDRATE	DIETARY FIBER	SUGARS	PROTEIN
2 g	57 mg	56 g	2 g	3 g	32 g

* FAT: EPA <1 g, DHA <1 g, ALA 0 g

Friday's Recipes

PAPAYA BANANA SALAD
YIELD: 4 CUPS

SERVES 4

2 cups papaya chunks
1 cup banana slices (about 2 small bananas)
1 cup chopped fresh navel orange
2 tablespoons orange juice

In a large bowl combine all the fruits and the juice. Let stand 30 minutes before serving.

NUTRITION PER 1-CUP SERVING

CALORIES	SODIUM	POTASSIUM	MAGNESIUM	CALCIUM	FAT*
83 kcal	3 mg	390 mg	22 mg	37 mg	<1 g

SATURATED FAT	CHOLESTEROL	CARBOHYDRATE	DIETARY FIBER	SUGARS	PROTEIN
<1 g	0 mg	21 g	3 g	13 g	1 g

* FAT: EPA 0 g, DHA 0 g, ALA 0 g

EGGLESS TOFU SALAD

YIELD: 2½ CUPS

SERVES 5

Serve on a bed of spinach or between 2 slices of whole-grain bread for a lunch rich in soy protein.

One 14-ounce container firm tofu
2 ribs celery, finely chopped (about ½ cup)
2 tablespoons minced onion
2 tablespoons light mayonnaise
1 tablespoon sweet pickle relish
1 teaspoon yellow prepared mustard
½ teaspoon dill weed
½ teaspoon turmeric
¼ teaspoon freshly ground black pepper

Crumble tofu into a colander and allow to drain for several minutes. Press with the back of a spoon to remove excess moisture, but leave the tofu in chunks so that it looks like chopped hard-cooked eggs. Dump the tofu into a bowl and mix with the remaining ingredients. Refrigerate until ready to serve. For best flavor chill several hours to allow flavors to blend.

NUTRITION PER ½-CUP SERVING

CALORIES	SODIUM	POTASSIUM	MAGNESIUM	CALCIUM	FAT*
85 kcal	106 mg	180 mg	33 mg	171 mg	5 g

SATURATED FAT	CHOLESTEROL	CARBOHYDRATE	DIETARY FIBER	SUGARS	PROTEIN
1 g	2 mg	4 g	1 g	1 g	7 g

* FAT: EPA 0 g, DHA 0 g, ALA 0 g

SLOW-COOKER TURKEY CHILI

YIELD: 10 CUPS

SERVES 8

I love to use the slow-cooker—it's a carefree way to have dinner ready whenever you are.

2 tablespoons olive oil

1 medium onion, peeled and chopped (about 1 cup)

1 large red bell pepper, seeded and chopped (about 1 cup)

4 cloves garlic, peeled and minced

2 tablespoons chili powder

2 tablespoons unsweetened cocoa powder

1 teaspoon ground cumin

2 teaspoons salt-free seasoning blend

½ teaspoon freshly ground black pepper

1 pound ground turkey breast

3 cups low-sodium vegetable juice

One 15-ounce can no-added-salt diced tomatoes with their juice

Two 15-ounce cans kidney beans, drained and rinsed

2 tablespoons molasses

2 avocados, peeled and diced

½ cup plain yogurt, divided

In a large skillet heat oil over medium heat. Add onion and bell pepper and cook until tender, about 5 minutes. Stir in the garlic, chili powder, cocoa powder, ground cumin, salt-free seasoning blend, and pepper. Cook for 1 minute to blend the spices. Pour onion and spice mixture in a slow cooker. Cook the turkey in the same skillet, breaking the turkey into small pieces and cooking until the turkey breast is no longer pink. Place in the slow cooker. Add the vegetable juice, tomatoes and their juice, kidney beans, and molasses. Cover the slow cooker and set on low power. Cook for 4 hours. Serve garnished with diced avocado and a spoonful of plain yogurt.

NUTRITION PER 1¼-CUP SERVING

CALORIES	SODIUM	POTASSIUM	MAGNESIUM	CALCIUM	FAT*
321 kcal	137 mg	1,217 mg	102 mg	141 mg	12 g

SATURATED FAT	CHOLESTEROL	CARBOHYDRATE	DIETARY FIBER	SUGARS	PROTEIN
2 g	36 mg	34 g	10 g	9 g	23 g

* FAT: EPA 0 g, DHA 0 g, ALA <1 g

Saturday's Recipes

DR. JANET'S SIMPLE ARUGULA SALAD

YIELD: 4 SERVINGS

Arugula, also known as rocket, is a highly nutritious leafy green vegetable of Mediterranean origin. A member of the brassica family, it is a cruciferous vegetable and a rich source of certain cancer-fighting phytochemicals such as indoles, thiocyanates, sulforaphane, and isothiocyanates.

> 10 ounces (2 bunches) fresh arugula
> Juice of one lemon
> 1 tablespoon white wine vinegar
> ¼ cup olive oil
> Dash of freshly ground black pepper
> 4 shavings Parmesan cheese

Remove ends of arugula, rinse, and pat dry. Add lemon juice and vinegar to a salad bowl. Whisk while drizzling in the olive oil. Add arugula and toss. Add pepper and top each serving with a shaving of cheese.

NUTRITION PER 1-CUP SERVING

CALORIES	SODIUM	POTASSIUM	MAGNESIUM	CALCIUM	FAT*
160 kcal	75 mg	267 mg	35 mg	156 mg	0 g

SATURATED FAT	CHOLESTEROL	CARBOHYDRATE	DIETARY FIBER	SUGARS	PROTEIN
<1 g	0 mg	2 g	1 g	2 g	3 g

* FAT: EPA 0 g, DHA 0 g, ALA 0 g

EASY SALMON CAKES

YIELD: 6 CAKES

SERVES 6

Traditional-style canned salmon contains bones. These can be easily mashed and blended into the fish for a rich addition of calcium.

> Two 14.75-ounce cans traditional-style pink salmon
> 2 scallions, thinly sliced
> ¼ cup finely chopped parsley
> 2 tablespoons Dijon mustard
> 2 tablespoons light mayonnaise
> ½ teaspoon salt-free seasoning blend
> 2 tablespoons canola oil

Place the salmon in a bowl. Use a large fork to flake the salmon and break up the skin and bones, mashing them into the salmon. Stir in the green onion, parsley, mustard, mayonnaise, and salt-free seasoning blend. Using a ½-cup measuring cup, portion out the salmon mixture into 6 portions. Shape each portion into a cake about 2 inches thick and 3 inches across. Chill for 1 hour. Heat oil in a heavy non-stick or cast-iron skillet. Cook cakes for 4 minutes on each side until golden brown on the outside and heated through. Keep warm until served.

NUTRITION PER CAKE

CALORIES	SODIUM	POTASSIUM	MAGNESIUM	CALCIUM	FAT*
207 kcal	709 mg	398 mg	40 mg	252 mg	12 g

SATURATED FAT	CHOLESTEROL	CARBOHYDRATE	DIETARY FIBER	SUGARS	PROTEIN
2 g	64 mg	1 g	<1 g	<1 g	23 g

* FAT: EPA 1 g, DHA 1 g, ALA 0 g

SHRIMP TACOS WITH KIWI SALSA

SERVES 4 (2 TACOS PER SERVING)

1 pound frozen cooked and peeled shrimp, thawed

¼ cup finely chopped red onion

¼ cup lime juice

2 cloves garlic, peeled and minced

1 teaspoon ground cumin

2 cups finely chopped kiwi (about 4 kiwi fruits)

¼ cup chopped fresh cilantro

¼ teaspoon crushed red pepper flakes

Eight 6-inch corn tortillas

1 avocado, peeled, pitted, and thinly sliced

In a large bowl, combine the cooked shrimp, red onion, lime juice, garlic, and ground cumin. In a medium bowl, combine kiwi, cilantro, and red pepper flakes. Cover both bowls with plastic wrap and refrigerate for at least 30 minutes, or preferably overnight.

Just before serving, heat the corn tortillas one at a time on a hot griddle until hot, about 15 seconds. Wrap the tortillas in a small towel and place in a basket to keep warm.

When ready to serve, divide the shrimp mixture among taco shells and top with the kiwi salsa. Serve with slices of avocado on top of the salsa.

(If you don't like shrimp, 1 pound of any firm-fleshed fish such as cod, halibut, or salmon can be used instead. First, cook the fish. Lightly brush the fillets with olive oil. Grill or sauté the fish on each side for about 4 minutes until done. Break the cooked fish into smaller chunks, and then proceed with the recipe.)

NUTRITION PER TACO

CALORIES	SODIUM	POTASSIUM	MAGNESIUM	CALCIUM	FAT*
167 kcal	148 mg	409 mg	48 mg	81 mg	5 g

SATURATED FAT	CHOLESTEROL	CARBOHYDRATE	DIETARY FIBER	SUGARS	PROTEIN
1 g	111 mg	19 g	4 g	4 g	14 g

* FAT: EPA <1 g, DHA <1 g, ALA <1 g

BLACK BEANS WITH SWEET POTATO

YIELD: 6 CUPS

SERVES 6

2 tablespoons olive oil

1 medium onion, peeled and chopped (about 1 cup)

1 large sweet potato, peeled and diced (about 2 cups)

4 cloves garlic, peeled and minced

1 teaspoon sweet paprika

1 teaspoon ground cumin

1 teaspoon dried oregano

1 teaspoon salt-free seasoning blend

⅛ teaspoon cayenne pepper, optional

Two 15-ounce cans black beans, drained and rinsed (about 3 cups)

1½ cups reduced-sodium chicken or vegetable broth

1 avocado, peeled and chopped for garnish

½ cup minced fresh cilantro for garnish

In a large skillet heat the oil over medium heat. Add the onion and sweet potato and cook for about 5 minutes until softened and lightly browned. Stir in the garlic, paprika, ground cumin, oregano, salt-free seasoning blend, and cayenne pepper. Cook for 30 seconds to soften the garlic, but be careful not to scorch the garlic or spices. Stir in the beans and chicken broth. Bring to a gentle boil, reduce heat to low, cover, and simmer for 20 minutes, stirring occasionally, until the sweet potatoes are soft. Uncover and cook for 10 more minutes to thicken the sauce. Garnish with chopped avocado and minced fresh cilantro if desired.

NUTRITION PER 1-CUP SERVING

CALORIES	SODIUM	POTASSIUM	MAGNESIUM	CALCIUM	FAT*
258 kcal	102 mg	711 mg	85 mg	60 mg	10 g

SATURATED FAT	CHOLESTEROL	CARBOHYDRATE	DIETARY FIBER	SUGARS	PROTEIN
1 g	0 mg	35 g	11 g	3 g	10 g

* FAT: EPA 0 g, DHA 0 g, ALA <1 g

SAUTÉED SPINACH WITH RAISINS AND PISTACHIOS

SERVES 4

One pound of fresh spinach sounds like a lot, but it cooks down to a manageable amount.

   1 tablespoon olive oil
   2 cloves garlic, peeled and minced
   ⅛ teaspoon crushed red pepper flakes
   1 pound fresh baby spinach (about 10 cups)
   ¼ cup raisins
   ½ teaspoon salt-free seasoning blend
   ¼ cup chopped pistachios

In a large skillet, heat oil over medium-low heat. Add the garlic and red pepper flakes and cook gently for 1 minute. Add the spinach and raisins. This is where you think you have too much spinach, but you don't. Using a pair of tongs, turn the spinach from underneath to the top and cook until wilted, about 2 minutes. Season with salt-free seasoning blend and top with chopped pistachios. Serve warm.

NUTRITION PER SERVING

CALORIES	SODIUM	POTASSIUM	MAGNESIUM	CALCIUM	FAT*
129 kcal	92 mg	788 mg	102 mg	128 mg	7 g

SATURATED FAT	CHOLESTEROL	CARBOHYDRATE	DIETARY FIBER	SUGARS	PROTEIN
1 g	0 mg	14 g	4 g	7 g	5 g

* FAT: EPA 0 g, DHA 0 g, ALA 0 g

Sunday's Recipes

SALMON BLACK BEAN QUESADILLAS

YIELD: 4 QUESADILLAS

Flour tortillas vary widely in sodium content. Fontova Foods makes a low-sodium, multigrain flour tortilla that has only 115 mg sodium per tortilla. Visit www.fontova.com for more information.

One 2.6-ounce pouch pink salmon
1 cup cooked black beans
1 cup frozen corn kernels, thawed
1 jalapeño pepper, seeded and chopped
¼ cup finely chopped red onion
¼ cup chopped fresh cilantro
Juice of one lime
Eight 8-inch Fontova multigrain flour tortillas
1 cup shredded part-skim mozzarella cheese
Nonstick cooking spray

In a large bowl stir together the salmon, black beans, corn, jalapeño, red onion, cilantro and lime juice. Lay 4 tortillas on a clean countertop. Sprinkle each tortilla with 2 tablespoons of shredded cheese. Top with ½ cup of the bean mixture. Sprinkle with another 2 tablespoons cheese. Top with the remaining tortilla and press down.

Preheat oven to 200°F. Spray a large nonstick skillet with cooking spray. Turn heat to medium-high and place 1 quesadilla in the skillet. Cook for about 4 minutes on each side or until golden brown and the cheese is melted and the filling is hot. Remove from the skillet to a baking sheet or large ovenproof platter and keep warm in the oven. With a paper towel wipe out the skillet and repeat the process for remaining quesadillas. Serve warm.

NUTRITION PER QUESADILLA

CALORIES	SODIUM	POTASSIUM	MAGNESIUM	CALCIUM	FAT*
264 kcal	190 mg	342 mg	50 mg	294 mg	0 g

SATURATED FAT	CHOLESTEROL	CARBOHYDRATE	DIETARY FIBER	SUGARS	PROTEIN
4 g	24 mg	35 g	7 g	3 g	15 g

* FAT: EPA <1 g, DHA <1 g, ALA 0 g

FRESH AVOCADO DIP (GUACAMOLE)

YIELD: 1 ½ CUPS

SERVES 6

Serve as a dip with low-salt bagel or pita chips, or as an accompaniment to the Salmon Black Bean Quesadillas (page 283) or Shrimp Tacos with Kiwi Salsa (page 280).

- 2 cups chopped avocado (from 2 medium avocados)
- ¼ cup chopped fresh cilantro
- 1 tablespoon lime juice
- ¼ teaspoon garlic powder
- ¼ teaspoon ground cumin
- ½ teaspoon salt-free seasoning blend
- 6 drops hot pepper sauce

Mash the avocado in a bowl with a fork until desired consistency. Mix in the cilantro, lime juice, garlic powder, ground cumin, salt-free seasoning blend, and hot pepper sauce. Serve immediately.

NUTRITION PER ¼-CUP SERVING

CALORIES	SODIUM	POTASSIUM	MAGNESIUM	CALCIUM	FAT*
98 kcal	6 mg	301 mg	17 mg	9 mg	9 g

SATURATED FAT	CHOLESTEROL	CARBOHYDRATE	DIETARY FIBER	SUGARS	PROTEIN
1 g	0 mg	5 g	4 g	<1 g	1 g

* FAT: EPA 0 g, DHA 0 g, ALA <1 g

WARM EDAMAME AND CORN SALAD

YIELD: 4 CUPS

SERVES 4

Frozen edamame is sold shelled or in the pod. For this recipe, use the shelled variety—it cooks quickly in the microwave and offers a soy-protein-rich alternative to lima beans in this twist on succotash.

2 cups frozen shelled edamame

1½ cups frozen corn kernels

1 red bell pepper, seeded and chopped

2 scallions, white part and some of the green part, thinly sliced

¼ cup chopped fresh basil

¼ cup olive oil

2 tablespoon red wine vinegar

1 clove garlic, peeled and minced

1 teaspoon Dijon mustard

½ teaspoon salt-free seasoning blend

½ teaspoon freshly ground black pepper

Place the edamame and corn in a microwave-safe dish. Add ¼ cup water. Place in microwave oven and cook on high power for 5 minutes, stirring once. Drain and mix in the chopped red pepper, green onion, and basil. Meanwhile, in another bowl whisk together the olive oil, red wine vinegar, garlic, Dijon mustard, salt-free seasoning blend, and pepper. Mix with the edamame mixture and serve warm.

NUTRITION PER 1-CUP SERVING

CALORIES	SODIUM	POTASSIUM	MAGNESIUM	CALCIUM	FAT*
314 kcal	34 mg	715 mg	74 mg	150 mg	20 g

SATURATED FAT	CHOLESTEROL	CARBOHYDRATE	DIETARY FIBER	SUGARS	PROTEIN
3 g	0 mg	26 g	6 g	3 g	14 g

* FAT: EPA 0 g, DHA 0 g, ALA 0 g

PENNE PASTA WITH LENTILS AND KALE

YIELD: 4 CUPS SAUCE

SERVES 8

If you like, fresh baby spinach can be substituted for the kale (reduce the final cooking time to 5 minutes).

- 3 tablespoons olive oil, divided
- 1 small onion, peeled and diced
- 2 carrots, peeled and diced
- ½ red bell pepper, seeded and chopped
- 2 cloves garlic, peeled and minced
- 1 teaspoon salt-free seasoning blend
- 1 teaspoon dried basil
- 1 teaspoon dried thyme
- ½ cup brown lentils, rinsed and picked over
- 3 cups low-sodium vegetable broth
- 8 ounces whole-grain penne pasta (about 2 cups dry)
- 1 pound fresh kale, tough stems removed, chopped (about 6 cups)
- 1 cup low-sodium vegetable juice
- ¼ teaspoon freshly ground black pepper

In a Dutch oven heat 2 tablespoons olive oil over medium heat. Add the onion, carrot, red pepper, and garlic. Cook until softened, about 8 minutes. Stir in the salt-free seasoning blend, basil, and thyme. Cook for 1 minute using caution not to scorch the herbs. Add the lentils and vegetable broth. Bring to a gentle boil and cover. Reduce heat to a simmer and cook for about 35 minutes or until lentils are tender.

Meanwhile, bring a large pot of water to a boil. Stir in the pasta and cook for 9 minutes or until desired degree of doneness.

When the lentils are tender stir in the kale and vegetable juice. Cover and cook for 15 minutes until the kale is tender but still a nice bright green. Serve the hot sauce over the pasta. Garnish with fresh black pepper and a drizzle of olive oil.

NUTRITION PER ½ CUP SAUCE AND 1 CUP PASTA SERVING

CALORIES	SODIUM	POTASSIUM	MAGNESIUM	CALCIUM	FAT*
238 kcal	150 mg	641 mg	81 mg	116 mg	6 g

SATURATED FAT	CHOLESTEROL	CARBOHYDRATE	DIETARY FIBER	SUGARS	PROTEIN
1 g	0 mg	39 g	6 g	2 g	11 g

* FAT: EPA 0 g, DHA 0 g, ALA 0 g

Week Two

Monday's Recipes

DR. JANET'S ROASTED TOFU AND CAULIFLOWER CURRY WITH BROWN RICE

SERVES 6

One 14-ounce container extra-firm tofu
One 2-pound head cauliflower, cut into 1-inch pieces (about 8 cups)
3 tablespoons olive oil
1 large sweet onion, halved and sliced
4 tablespoons curry powder
1 teaspoon ground ginger
1 teaspoon ground cumin
1 teaspoon salt-free seasoning blend
3 cups cooked brown rice.

Preheat oven to 450°F. Remove tofu from the container and drain. Place several paper towels on a plate. Set the tofu on the paper towels and put several more paper towels on top of the tofu. Place a heavy plate on top of the tofu to press the excess moisture out of the tofu. Cut the tofu into 1-inch pieces and combine with the cauliflower. Set aside.

In a large skillet heat the oil over medium heat. Add the onion, and cook, stirring until golden brown, about 5 minutes. Stir in the curry, ginger, ground cumin, and salt-free seasoning blend, to coat the onions. Mix the curry and onion mixture with the cauliflower and tofu. Stir gently to combine. Spray a baking sheet with nonstick cooking spray. Spread the tofu and cauliflower in a single layer on the sheet and bake, stirring occasionally, for about 30 minutes or until the cauliflower is tender. Serve over cooked brown rice.

NUTRITION PER 1 CUP CAULIFLOWER AND ½ CUP BROWN RICE

CALORIES	SODIUM	POTASSIUM	MAGNESIUM	CALCIUM	FAT*
279 kcal	62 mg	709 mg	104 mg	205 mg	11 g

SATURATED FAT	CHOLESTEROL	CARBOHYDRATE	DIETARY FIBER	SUGARS	PROTEIN
2 g	0 mg	37 g	8 g	6 g	12 g

* FAT: EPA 0 g, DHA 0 g, ALA 0 g

Tuesday's Recipes

ROASTED VEGETABLES WITH QUINOA AND SPINACH

YIELD: 8 CUPS

SERVES 8

Can be served as a side dish or an entrée. Be sure to rinse the quinoa before cooking.

- 1 pound carrots, peeled and cut into 1½-inch lengths
- 1 pound portobello mushroom caps, stems removed and cut into 1½-inch chunks
- 3 tablespoons olive oil, divided
- 1 teaspoon salt-free seasoning blend
- ½ teaspoon black pepper
- 5 cups fresh baby spinach (about 8 ounces)
- 2 tablespoons fresh lemon juice
- 2 tablespoons fresh thyme leaves
- ½ cup quinoa
- ¼ cup chopped pistachios

Preheat oven to 425° F. On a baking sheet toss the carrots and mushrooms with 2 tablespoons olive oil, salt-free seasoning blend, and pepper. Place in the oven and cook, mixing once, until tender, about 20 to 25 minutes. Remove the vegetables from the baking sheet to a large bowl. Toss with the spinach, lemon juice, and thyme.

Meanwhile, rinse quinoa in a sieve. Place rinsed quinoa and 1 cup water in a saucepan. Bring to a boil, reduce heat to low, cover and cook for 15 minutes. Remove from the heat and let sit for 5 minutes. Fluff the quinoa with a fork and toss with the spinach and roasted vegetables. Sprinkle with the pistachios and drizzle with the remaining 1 tablespoon of olive oil.

NUTRITION PER 1-CUP SERVING

CALORIES	SODIUM	POTASSIUM	MAGNESIUM	CALCIUM	FAT*
151 kcal	60 mg	689 mg	56 mg	56 mg	7 g

SATURATED FAT	CHOLESTEROL	CARBOHYDRATE	DIETARY FIBER	SUGARS	PROTEIN
1 g	0 mg	18 g	4 g	4 g	5 g

* FAT: EPA 0 g, DHA 0 g, ALA 0 g

Wednesday's Recipes

LENTIL AND TEMPEH STEW

YIELD: 12 CUPS

SERVES 12

Build the flavor in this stew by letting the onions cook until golden brown.

2 tablespoons olive oil
1 large onion, peeled and chopped
One 8-ounce package soy tempeh, cut into 1-inch chunks
4 cloves garlic, peeled and minced
2 teaspoons curry powder
¼ teaspoon ground cinnamon
¼ teaspoon ground ginger
2 cups brown lentils, picked over and rinsed
1 pound sweet potatoes, peeled and cut into ½-inch chunks
One 14½ ounce can no-added-salt diced tomatoes (about 1½ cups)
4 cups water
3 cups low-sodium vegetable broth
2 teaspoons salt-free seasoning blend
½ teaspoon freshly ground black pepper
Juice of one lemon
4 ounces fresh baby spinach (about 3 cups)

In a Dutch oven heat oil over medium heat. Add onion and cook for about 8 minutes, until golden brown. Stir in the diced tempeh, garlic, curry powder, cinnamon, and ginger. Cook, stirring for 2 minutes to coat the tempeh with the spices. Add the lentils, sweet potatoes, tomatoes, water, broth, salt-free seasoning blend, and pepper. Bring to a boil. Reduce heat to a simmer, cover, and cook for about 45 to 50 minutes until lentils are cooked through. Stir in the lemon juice and baby spinach and cook until the spinach is wilted, about 5 minutes.

NUTRITION PER 1-CUP SERVING

CALORIES	SODIUM	POTASSIUM	MAGNESIUM	CALCIUM	FAT*
219 kcal	110 mg	698 mg	73 mg	78 mg	5 g

SATURATED FAT	CHOLESTEROL	CARBOHYDRATE	DIETARY FIBER	SUGARS	PROTEIN
1 g	0 mg	32 g	12 g	4 g	15 g

* FAT: EPA 0 g, DHA 0 g, ALA 0 g

Thursday's Recipes

APRICOT AND ALMOND BUCKWHEAT PILAF

YIELD: 4 CUPS

SERVES 4

Look for kasha (100 percent pure roasted whole-grain buckwheat) in the kosher section of a large supermarket. I like Wolff's brand. Bulk-purchased whole-grain buckwheat can also be used (but you will need to toast it before cooking).

> 1 tablespoon olive oil
> 1 small onion, peeled and diced
> 1 cup kasha or whole-grain buckwheat
> ½ cup sliced almonds
> 12 apricot halves, cut into small pieces with a pair of kitchen shears
> ½ teaspoon salt-free seasoning blend
> ¼ teaspoon freshly ground black pepper
> 2 cups low-sodium vegetable broth

In a large skillet heat the olive oil over medium heat. Add the onion and cook for about 5 minutes until golden brown. Stir in the kasha, almonds, apricots, salt-free seasoning and pepper. Stir until the kasha is coated with the oil and the almonds are slightly toasted, about 1 minute. Carefully add the broth and bring to a gentle boil. Cover, reduce heat to a simmer, and cook for 15 minutes. Remove from the heat and let sit 5 minutes. Fluff with a fork before serving.

NUTRITION PER 1-CUP SERVING

CALORIES	SODIUM	POTASSIUM	MAGNESIUM	CALCIUM	FAT*
339 kcal	151 mg	466 mg	129 mg	55 mg	17 g

SATURATED FAT	CHOLESTEROL	CARBOHYDRATE	DIETARY FIBER	SUGARS	PROTEIN
2 g	0 mg	42 g	6 g	7 g	9 g

* FAT: EPA 0 g, DHA 0 g, ALA 0 g

Friday's Recipes

FRUIT SALAD WITH POPPY SEED YOGURT DRESSING

YIELD: 8 CUPS

SERVES 8

½ cup plain low-fat yogurt
1 tablespoon honey
1 tablespoon lemon juice
1 tablespoon olive oil
1 teaspoon poppy seeds
4 cups diced cantaloupe (from about 1 medium-sized cantaloupe)
1 cup diced kiwi (from about 2 kiwi)
1 cup sliced strawberries
2 cups banana, sliced (2 medium bananas)

In a large bowl whisk together the yogurt, honey, lemon juice, olive oil, and poppy seeds. Gently fold in the chopped fruit. Add the bananas just before serving.

NUTRITION PER 1-CUP SERVING

CALORIES	SODIUM	POTASSIUM	MAGNESIUM	CALCIUM	FAT*
115 kcal	23 mg	485 mg	30 mg	53 mg	3 g

SATURATED FAT	CHOLESTEROL	CARBOHYDRATE	DIETARY FIBER	SUGARS	PROTEIN
<1 g	1 mg	23 g	3 g	17 g	2 g

* FAT: EPA 0 g, DHA 0 g, ALA 0 g

CREAMY CANNELLINI BEAN WITH SPINACH SOUP

YIELD: 6 CUPS

SERVES 6

Canned white cannellini beans are an excellent source of potassium and make a quick soup.

1 tablespoon olive oil

1 medium onion, peeled and finely chopped (about 1 cup)

1 rib celery, finely chopped

4 cloves garlic, peeled and minced

Two 15-ounce cans cannellini beans, drained and rinsed

3 cups low-sodium chicken broth

¼ teaspoon dried thyme

1 teaspoon salt-free seasoning blend

¼ teaspoon finely ground black pepper

5 ounces fresh baby spinach (about 4 cups)

1 tablespoon fresh lemon juice

In a saucepan heat the oil over medium heat. Add the onion and celery and cook stirring until tender, about 5 minutes. Add garlic and stir for 1 minute. Add beans, broth, thyme, salt-free seasoning blend, and pepper; blend. Bring to a boil, reduce heat to a simmer, and cook uncovered for 15 minutes. With the back of a large spoon smash the beans up against the side of the pot to thicken the soup. Pick through the baby spinach to remove any large stems or discolored leaves. Stir the spinach into the soup and cook for about 2 minutes or until the spinach is reduced in size and wilted into the soup. Stir in the lemon juice. Serve with more freshly ground black pepper if desired.

NUTRITION PER 1-CUP SERVING

CALORIES	SODIUM	POTASSIUM	MAGNESIUM	CALCIUM	FAT*
169 kcal	171 mg	785 mg	79 mg	124 mg	3 g

SATURATED FAT	CHOLESTEROL	CARBOHYDRATE	DIETARY FIBER	SUGARS	PROTEIN
<1 g	0 mg	27 g	6 g	1 g	11 g

* FAT: EPA 0 g, DHA 0 g, ALA 0 g

WARM HERBED POTATO SALAD

SERVES 8

2 pounds small red potatoes (about 15), halved

¼ cup chopped fresh flat-leaf parsley

¼ cup chopped fresh dill

2 scallions thinly sliced

2 tablespoons olive oil

1 tablespoon whole-grain mustard

1 tablespoon red wine vinegar

½ teaspoon salt-free seasoning blend

¼ teaspoon freshly ground black pepper

Place potatoes in a saucepan and cover with cold water. Bring to a boil and cook for 20 minutes or until tender. Drain. Meanwhile, in a medium bowl, mix together the parsley, dill, green onion, oil, mustard, vinegar, salt-free seasoning blend, and pepper. Add the warm cooked potatoes and blend to combine. Serve warm or at room temperature.

NUTRITION PER SERVING

CALORIES	SODIUM	POTASSIUM	MAGNESIUM	CALCIUM	FAT*
116 kcal	33 mg	544 mg	27 mg	20 mg	4 g

SATURATED FAT	CHOLESTEROL	CARBOHYDRATE	DIETARY FIBER	SUGARS	PROTEIN
<1 g	0 mg	19 g	2 g	1 g	2 g

* FAT: EPA 0 g, DHA 0 g, ALA 0 g

ALMOND THUMBPRINT COOKIES

YIELD: ABOUT TWENTY 2-INCH COOKIES

This hearty cookie is filled with apricot fruit spread, but you can use raspberry or strawberry fruit spread, too.

> 1 cup whole almonds
> 2 cups quick-cooking oats
> ½ cup all-purpose flour, plus 2 tablespoons if needed
> ½ cup canola oil
> 2 tablespoons pure maple syrup
> ⅓ cup plus 1 tablespoon molasses
> ½ cup apricot all-fruit spread

In a food processor pulse the almonds for 45 seconds until gritty like sand. Add the oats and pulse for 30 more seconds to grind the almonds and oats together. Add ½ cup flour and pulse to mix. Pour in the oil, maple syrup, and molasses. Mix in the food processor until well combined. If the dough seems too wet (it will be sticky, but should not be runny) add the additional 2 tablespoons flour. Dump the dough into a bowl, cover, and let sit for 10 minutes. Meanwhile, cover 2 baking sheets with parchment paper. Using your hands or a small scoop form the dough into balls the size of a small walnut and place on the cookie sheet. Using the back of a small spoon, or your thumb, make a small indentation in each cookie. Fill the indentation with ½ teaspoon of the apricot fruit spread. Bake for 15 minutes or until the cookies start to brown slightly. Do not overcook or the cookies will become too hard when cooled. Let the cookies cool on the pan for 15 minutes; then move them to a rack to cool completely. Store in an airtight container.

NUTRITION PER COOKIE

CALORIES	SODIUM	POTASSIUM	MAGNESIUM	CALCIUM	FAT*
150 kcal	5 mg	199 mg	41 mg	31 mg	8 g

SATURATED FAT	CHOLESTEROL	CARBOHYDRATE	DIETARY FIBER	SUGARS	PROTEIN
1 g	0 mg	18 g	2 g	5 g	2 g

* FAT: EPA 0 g, DHA 0 g, ALA 0 g

Saturday's Recipes

DR. JANET'S ROASTED SWEET POTATO FRIES

SERVES 4

Bake in the oven for a fresh, potassium-filled side dish.

- 4 small sweet potatoes, scrubbed and dried (about 1½ pounds)
- 3 tablespoons olive oil
- 1 teaspoon salt-free seasoning blend
- ¼ cup minced fresh rosemary (from one small bunch)

Preheat oven to 425°F. Cover a large baking sheet with aluminum foil. Halve potatoes lengthwise and then cut each piece in half again into 4 wedges and place in a large bowl. Toss with oil, salt-free seasoning blend, and rosemary. Place potatoes on baking sheet in a single layer, cut-side of potatoes down. Bake for 15 minutes. With tongs turn the potatoes over to place the other cut-side down. Return to the oven and bake for 15 minutes more. Serve immediately.

NUTRITION PER 8 FRIES

CALORIES	SODIUM	POTASSIUM	MAGNESIUM	CALCIUM	FAT*
238 kcal	94 mg	585 mg	44 mg	57 mg	10 g

SATURATED FAT	CHOLESTEROL	CARBOHYDRATE	DIETARY FIBER	SUGARS	PROTEIN
1 g	0 mg	35 g	5 g	7 g	3 g

* FAT: EPA 0 g, DHA 0 g, ALA 0 g

CHOCOLATE BANANA CAKE

SERVES 18

2 cups all-purpose flour
½ cup Splenda Brown Sugar Blend
¼ cup unsweetened cocoa powder
½ teaspoon baking soda
1 large ripe banana, mashed (½ cup)
¾ cup soy milk
¼ cup canola oil
1 large egg
1 egg white
1 tablespoon lemon juice
1 teaspoon vanilla extract
½ cup semisweet chocolate chips

Preheat oven to 350°F. Spray an 11-by-7-inch brownie pan with nonstick spray. Whisk together flour, sugar blend, cocoa, and baking soda in large bowl. In another bowl whisk together the banana, soy milk, oil, egg, egg white, lemon juice, and vanilla. Make a hole in the middle of the flour mixture and pour on the soy milk mixture and chocolate chips. With a wooden spoon stir the ingredients together until blended. Spoon batter into pan. Bake about 25 minutes until the center of the cake springs back when pressed lightly with fingertips.

NUTRITION PER SERVING

CALORIES	SODIUM	POTASSIUM	MAGNESIUM	CALCIUM	FAT[*]
150 kcal	52 mg	119 mg	19 mg	23 mg	4 g

SATURATED FAT	CHOLESTEROL	CARBOHYDRATE	DIETARY FIBER	SUGARS	PROTEIN
1 g	12 mg	27 g	1 g	9 g	3 g

* FAT: EPA 0 g, DHA 0 g, ALA 0 g

Bonus Recipes

BAKED SWEET POTATO WITH CINNAMON YOGURT TOPPING

YIELD: 4

SERVES 4

- 4 medium sweet potatoes (about 8 ounces each)
- ½ cup vanilla nonfat yogurt
- ¼ teaspoon cinnamon
- 8 dried apricot halves, slivered
- 2 tablespoons chopped walnuts

Preheat oven to 400°F. Poke the surface of the potatoes several times with a fork; then place them on a baking sheet. Bake for about 50 to 55 minutes or until easily pierced with a fork. Meanwhile, in a separate bowl, whisk together the yogurt, cinnamon, apricots, and walnuts. Just before serving use a knife to cut a slit in the top of each potato. Pull the potatoes open to expose the cooked flesh and spoon 2 tablespoons of yogurt topping onto each potato.

NUTRITION PER POTATO WITH 2 TABLESPOONS YOGURT TOPPING

CALORIES	SODIUM	POTASSIUM	MAGNESIUM	CALCIUM	FAT[*]
178 kcal	93 mg	603 mg	43 mg	100 mg	3 g

SATURATED FAT	CHOLESTEROL	CARBOHYDRATE	DIETARY FIBER	SUGARS	PROTEIN
<1 g	2 mg	35 g	5 g	14 g	4 g

[*] FAT: EPA 0 g, DHA 0 g, ALA 0 g

CORN AND ARTICHOKE SALAD WITH BASIL DRESSING

YIELD: 5½ CUPS

SERVES 11

1 cup frozen corn kernels, thawed

One 14-ounce can quartered artichoke hearts, drained and sliced

One 15-ounce can cannellini beans, drained and rinsed (about
     1½ cups)

1 medium Hass avocado, peeled, pitted, and diced

½ red bell pepper, seeded and diced (about ½ cup)

1 small clove garlic, crushed

1 tablespoon honey

Juice of half a lemon (about 1 tablespoon)

2 tablespoons olive oil

½ teaspoon dried basil

½ teaspoon salt-free seasoning blend

In a bowl gently mix the corn, artichoke hearts, cannellini beans, avocado, and red pepper. Place the garlic, honey, lemon juice, olive oil, basil, and salt-free seasoning blend in a blender. Pulse to blend all ingredients until smooth. Toss the dressing with the salad ingredients. Serve immediately.

NUTRITION PER ½-CUP SERVING

CALORIES	SODIUM	POTASSIUM	MAGNESIUM	CALCIUM	FAT*
114 kcal	78 mg	342 mg	37 mg	36 mg	5 g

SATURATED FAT	CHOLESTEROL	CARBOHYDRATE	DIETARY FIBER	SUGARS	PROTEIN
5 g	0 mg	15 g	4 g	3 g	4 g

* FAT: EPA 0 g, DHA 0 g, ALA <1 g

EDAMAME HUMMUS

SERVES 8

Fresh green soybeans (edamame) serve as the base for this garlicky and spicy dip. Serve with sliced fresh vegetables.

2 cups frozen shelled edamame (one 12-ounce package)
¼ cup tahini
3 cloves garlic, peeled
Juice of two lemons (about ¼ cup)
2 tablespoons olive oil
1 teaspoon ground cumin
½ teaspoon salt-free seasoning blend
¼ teaspoon cayenne pepper
½ cup water

Place edamame in a microwave-safe dish. Cover with plastic wrap and cook on high for 3 minutes. Remove from microwave, drain, and let cool.

In a food processor combine the edamame, tahini, garlic, lemon juice, oil, ground cumin, salt-free seasoning, cayenne pepper, and water. Process for 1 minute, until smooth. Scrape down the sides and process for an additional 30 seconds. Store refrigerated.

NUTRITION PER ¼-CUP SERVING

CALORIES	SODIUM	POTASSIUM	MAGNESIUM	CALCIUM	FAT*
144 kcal	10 mg	302 mg	36 mg	82 mg	10 g

SATURATED FAT	CHOLESTEROL	CARBOHYDRATE	DIETARY FIBER	SUGARS	PROTEIN
<1 g	0 mg	8 g	2 g	<1 g	8 g

* FAT: EPA 0 g, DHA 0 g, ALA 0 g

SWEET POTATO BROWN RICE

YIELD: 6 CUPS

SERVES 6

2 tablespoons olive oil
1 cup chopped yellow onion
1 cup long-grain brown rice
½ cup sliced almonds
1 teaspoon cumin
1 teaspoon salt-free seasoning blend
¼ teaspoon freshly ground black pepper
2 cups water
1 medium sweet potato, peeled and cut into ½-inch pieces

In a large skillet with a lid, heat oil over medium heat. Add the onion and cook stirring occasionally until golden brown, about 5 minutes. Add the rice, almonds, cumin, salt-free seasoning blend, and pepper and stir for about 1 minute to toast the almonds and rice, but use caution not to burn the spices. Add the water and bring to a boil. Cover and reduce heat to a simmer and cook for 25 minutes. Remove the lid and scatter the sweet potatoes over the rice. Cover and cook for 20 more minutes or until the potatoes are tender. Remove from the heat and let sit for 5 minutes. Fluff with a fork before serving.

NUTRITION PER 1-CUP SERVING

CALORIES	SODIUM	POTASSIUM	MAGNESIUM	CALCIUM	FAT*
249 kcal	28 mg	319 mg	80 mg	549 mg	9 g

SATURATED FAT	CHOLESTEROL	CARBOHYDRATE	DIETARY FIBER	SUGARS	PROTEIN
1 g	0 mg	37 g	4 g	4 g	5 g

* FAT: EPA 0 g, DHA 0 g, ALA 0 g

QUINOA PILAF WITH RAISINS AND PEAS

YIELD: 6 CUPS

SERVES 6

An easy alternative to rice pilaf. Be sure to rinse the quinoa before cooking.

1 cup quinoa
2 tablespoons olive oil
1 cup thinly sliced yellow onion
1 teaspoon ground cumin
¼ teaspoon cinnamon
¼ teaspoon ground cardamom
½ cup sliced almonds
2½ cups water
¼ cup dark raisins
1 teaspoon salt-free seasoning blend
¼ teaspoon freshly ground black pepper
1½ cups frozen green peas

Rinse quinoa in a sieve with cool running water. Let drain and set aside.

In a skillet with a lid, heat oil over medium heat. Add the onion and cook, stirring occasionally until golden brown. Add the ground cumin, cinnamon, cardamom, and almonds. Stir to combine with the onions for about 30 seconds, using caution not to burn the spices. Add the rinsed and drained quinoa and cook, stirring for about 1 minute to toast the quinoa, again using caution not to burn the spices. Add the water, raisins, salt-free seasoning, and pepper. Bring to a boil. Cover and reduce heat to low. Cook for 15 minutes. Add the peas on top of the quinoa without stirring. Cover and cook for 5 more minutes. Remove from the heat and leave covered for 10 more minutes. Fluff with a fork before serving.

NUTRITION PER 1-CUP SERVING

CALORIES	SODIUM	POTASSIUM	MAGNESIUM	CALCIUM	FAT*
249 kcal	49 mg	406 mg	96 mg	70 mg	10 g

SATURATED FAT	CHOLESTEROL	CARBOHYDRATE	DIETARY FIBER	SUGARS	PROTEIN
1 g	0 mg	34 g	5 g	7 g	7 g

* FAT: EPA 0 g, DHA 0 g, ALA 0 g

SWISS CHARD AND WHITE BEAN STEW

YIELD: 8 CUPS

SERVES 8

The Swiss chard shrinks as it cooks, so don't be alarmed at the amount that goes into the pot.

> 2 tablespoons olive oil
> 4 cloves garlic, sliced
> ¼ teaspoon crushed red pepper flakes
> One 28-ounce can no-added-salt diced tomatoes with their juice
> ¼ cup dry red wine
> 1 teaspoon dried basil
> 1 teaspoon salt-free seasoning blend
> ½ teaspoon dried thyme
> 1½ pounds Swiss chard, large stems discarded and leaves cut into
>   1-inch pieces
> Two 15-ounce cans cannellini beans, drained and rinsed (about 3 cups)
> About 2 tablespoons olive oil, for drizzling
> ½ teaspoon freshly ground black pepper

In a Dutch oven or soup pot heat the oil over medium-low heat. Add the garlic and crushed red pepper flakes and cook gently until garlic is golden, about 2 minutes. Add the tomatoes, red wine, basil, thyme, and salt-free seasoning blend. Bring to a simmer and cook for about 15 minutes to blend the flavors and reduce the wine. Stir in the chopped chard, cover, and simmer for an additional 10 minutes until the chard is tender. Stir in the beans and cook, covered, for 10 more minutes to blend flavors and heat the beans. Serve in bowls drizzled with olive oil and freshly ground black pepper.

NUTRITION PER 1-CUP SERVING

CALORIES	SODIUM	POTASSIUM	MAGNESIUM	CALCIUM	FAT[*]
195 kcal	197 mg	926 mg	124 mg	136 mg	7 g

SATURATED FAT	CHOLESTEROL	CARBOHYDRATE	DIETARY FIBER	SUGARS	PROTEIN
1 g	0 mg	25 g	7 g	1 g	9 g

* FAT: EPA 0 g, DHA 0 g, ALA 0 g

SAM'S DARK CHOCOLATE ALMOND BARK

SERVES 16

A sinfully rich and satisfying dark chocolate treat. Perfect savored with a glass of red wine or a cup of green tea for a powerful blood-pressure-lowering dessert cocktail!

> **12 ounces (12 squares) Baker's unsweetened baking chocolate squares**
> **6 tablespoons Splenda® Sugar Blend for baking**
> **1 cup unsalted, dry roasted almonds**

Place chocolate squares in a double boiler and melt until creamy. Add the sugar and continue stirring until smooth. Remove pot from the heat and stir in the almonds. Make sure the almonds are completely covered with the chocolate. Line a cookie sheet with parchment paper and spread the almond mixture evenly on the parchment into a thin layer, spacing almonds evenly. Chill the bark in the refrigerator for approximately 1 hour until firm. Remove, break into small pieces, and enjoy!

NUTRITION PER ¹⁄₁₆ OF ALMOND BARK (A LITTLE OVER AN OUNCE IN WEIGHT)

CALORIES	SODIUM	POTASSIUM	MAGNESIUM	CALCIUM	FAT*
170 kcal	0 mg	65 mg	25 mg	23 mg	15 g

SATURATED FAT	CHOLESTEROL	CARBOHYDRATE	DIETARY FIBER	SUGARS	PROTEIN
7 g	0 mg	10 g	4 g	3 g	5 g

* FAT: EPA 0 g, DHA 0 g, ALA 0 g

Notes

Introduction

1. Danaei G, Ding EL, Mozaffarian D, et al. The preventable causes of death in the United States: comparative risk assessment of dietary, lifestyle, and metabolic risk factors. *PLoS Med* 2009:6(4):e1000058. DOI:10.1371/journal.pmed.1000058.

Chapter One. Understanding the Problem

1. Kones R. Primary prevention of coronary heart disease: integration of new data, evolving views, revised goals, and role of rosuvastatin in management. A comprehensive survey. *Drug Des Devel Ther* 2011;5:325–380.

2. Heidenreich PA, Trogdon JG, Khavjou OA, et al. Forecasting the future of cardiovascular disease in the United States: a policy statement from the American Heart Association. *Circulation* 2011;123:933–944.

3. Roger VL, Go AS, Lloyd-Jones DM, Benjamin EJ, et al., on behalf of the American Heart Association Statistics Committee and Stroke Statistics Subcommittee. Heart disease and stroke statistics—2012 update: a report from the American Heart Association. *Circulation* 2012;125:e2–e220.

4. Gaziano TA, et al. The global cost of nonoptimal blood pressure. *J Hypertens* 2009;27:1472–1477.

5. Sheltens T, et al. Awareness of hypertension: will it bring about a healthy lifestyle? *J Hum Hypertens* 2010;24:561–567.

6. National High Blood Pressure Education Program. The seventh report of the Joint National Committee on Prevention, Detec-

tion, Evaluation, and Treatment of High Blood Pressure. *Hypertens* 2003;42:1206–1252.

7. Pickering TG, et al. Recommendations for blood pressure measurement in humans and experimental animals. Part 1: Blood pressure measurement in humans: a statement for professionals from the Subcommittee of Professional and Public Education of the American Heart Association Council on High Blood Pressure Research. *Hypertens* 2005;45:142–161.

8. Clark CE, Powell RJ. The differential blood pressure sign in general practice: prevalence and prognostic value. *Family Practice* 2002; 19:439–441.

9. Pickering TG, et al. Recommendations for blood pressure measurement in humans and experimental animals. Part 1: Blood pressure measurement in humans.

Chapter Two. High Blood Pressure: The Silent Killer

1. National Heart Lung and Blood Institute. What is heart failure? www .nhlbi.nih.gov/health/health-topics/topics/hf/

2. Furberg CD. Renin-guided treatment of hypertension: time for action. *Am J Hypertens* 2010;23(9):929–930.

3. Jones DW, Miller ME, Wofford MR, et al. The effect of weight loss intervention on antihypertensive medication requirements in the Hypertension Optimal Treatment (HOT) study. *Am J Hypertens* 1999;12:1175–1180.

Chapter Three. Blood Pressure Down: A Potent Natural Combination Therapy

1. Sever PS, Messerli FH. Hypertension management 2011: optimal combination therapy. *Eur Heart J* 2011;32:2499–2506.

2. Chobanian AV, Bakris GL, Black HR, et al. The seventh report of the Joint National Committee on Prevention, Detection, Evaluation, and Treatment of High Blood Pressure: the JNC 7 report. *JAMA* 2003;289(19):2560–2571.

3. Ibid.

4. Whelton PK, He J, Appel LJ, et al., for the National High Blood Pressure Education Program Coordinating Committee. Primary prevention of hypertension: clinical and public health advisory from the National High Blood Pressure Education Program. *JAMA* 2002;288(15):1882–1888.

5. Appel LJ, Brands MW, Daniels SR, et al. Dietary approaches to prevent and treat hypertension: a scientific statement from the American Heart Association. *Hypertens* 2006;47:296–308.

6. Khan N, Hemmelgarn B, Padwal R, et al. The 2009 Canadian Hypertension Education Program recommendations for the management of hypertension: part 2—therapy. *Can J Cardiol* 2009;25(5):287–298.

7. Williams B, Poulter NR, Brown MJ, et al. Guidelines for management of hypertension: report of the fourth working party of the British Hypertension Society, 2004—BHS IV. *J Hum Hypertens* 2004;18:139–185.

8. Blumenthal JA, Babyak MA, Hinderliter A, Watkins LL, Craighead L, Lin P-H, et al. Effects of the DASH diet alone and in combination with exercise and weight loss on blood pressure and cardiovascular biomarkers in men and women with high blood pressure: the ENCORE study. *Arch Int Med* 2010;170(2):126–135.

9. Cox KL, Puddey IB, Morton AR, et al. Exercise and weight control in sedentary overweight men: effects on clinic and ambulatory blood pressure. *J Hypertens* 1996;14:779–790.

10. Whelton PK, Appel LJ, Espeland MA, et al., for the TONE Collaborative Research Group. Sodium reduction and weight loss in the treatment of hypertension in older persons: a randomized controlled trial of nonpharmacologic interventions in the elderly (TONE). *JAMA* 1998;279(11):839–846.

11. Chobanian AV, Bakris GL, Black HR, et al. The seventh report of the Joint National Committee on Prevention, Detection, Evaluation, and Treatment of High Blood Pressure.

Chapter Four. Step 1: Lose Five Pounds

1. World Health Organization. Global health Risks: mortality and burden of disease attributable to selected major risks. www.who.int/healthinfo/global_burden_disease/GlobalHealthRisks_report_full.pdf

2. Masuo K, Mikami H, Ogihara T, Tuck ML. Weight reduction and pharmacologic treatment in obese hypertensives. *Am J Hypertens* 2001;14:530–538.

3. Fogari R, Zoppi A, Corradi L, Preti P, Mugellini A, Lazzari P, Derosa G. Effect of body weight loss and normalization on blood pressure in overweight non-obese patients with stage 1 hypertension. *Hypertens Res* 2010. Mar;33(3):236–242; Masuo K, Mikami H, Ogihara T, Tuck ML. Weight reduction and pharmacologic treatment in obese hypertensives.

4. Chobanian AV, Bakris GL, Black HR, et al. The seventh report of the Joint National Committee on Prevention, Detection, Evaluation, and Treatment of High Blood Pressure: the JNC 7 report. *JAMA* 2003;289(19):2560–2571.

5. Forman JP, Stampfer MJ, Curhan GC. Diet and lifestyle risk factors associated with incident hypertension in women. *JAMA* 2009;302(4):401–411.

6. Ibid.

7. Mozaffarian D, Tao H, Rimm EB, et al. Changes in diet and lifestyle and long-term weight gain in women and men. *N Eng J Med* 2011;364:2392–2404.

8. Aucott L, Rothnie H, McIntyre L, Thapa M, Waweru C, Gray D. Long-term weight loss from lifestyle intervention benefits blood pressure? A systematic review. *Hypertens* 2009;54:756–762.

9. Neter JE, Stam BE, Kok FJ, Grobbee DE, Geleijnse JM. Influence of weight reduction on blood pressure: a meta-analysis of randomized controlled trials. *Hypertens* 2003;42:878–884.

10. Aucott L, Rothnie H, McIntyre L, Thapa M, Waweru C, Gray D. Long-term weight loss from lifestyle intervention benefits blood pressure?

11. Neter JE, Stam BE, Kok FJ, Grobbee DE, Geleijnse JM. Influence of weight reduction on blood pressure.

12. Trials of Hypertension Prevention Collaborative Research Group. The effects of non-pharmacological interventions on blood pressure of persons with high normal levels: results of the Trials of Hypertension Prevention (Phase I). *JAMA* 1992;267:1213–1220.

13. Kruger J, Serdula MK, Jones DA. Attempting to lose weight: specific practices among US adults. *Amer J Prev Med* 2004;26(5):402–406.

14. Sacks FM, et al. Comparison of weight-loss diets with different compositions of fat, protein, and carbohydrates. *New Eng J Med* 2009;360(9):859–873.

15. Rolls BJ, Hetherington M, Burley VJ. The specificity of satiety: the influence of foods of different macronutrient content on the development of satiety. *Physiol Behav* 1988;43(2):145–153.

16. Qi BB, Dennis KE. The adoption of eating behaviors conducive to weight loss. *Eat Behav* 2000;1(1):23–31.

17. Butryn ML, Phelan S, Hill JO, Wing RR. Consistent self monitoring of weight: a key component of successful weight loss maintenance. *Obesity* 2007;15(12):3091–3096.

18. Donnelly JE, et al. American College of Sports Medicine position stand: appropriate physical activity intervention strategies for weight loss and prevention of weight regain for adults. *Med Sci Sports Exerc* 2009;41(2):459–471.

19. University of Texas M. D. Anderson Cancer Center. Obesity reversed in mice by destroying blood vessels that service fat cells. *ScienceDaily* 2004. May 10.

20. Schillaci G, Pirro M. Long-term weight loss and blood pressure reduction: the perfect is the enemy of the good. *Am J Hypertens* 2006;19(11):1101–1102.

Chapter Five. Step 2: Cut the Salt

1. Centers for Disease Control and Prevention. Where's the sodium? There's too much in many common foods. *CDC Vital Signs, February 2012*. www.cdc.gov/VitalSigns/Sodium/index.html

2. MacGregor G, de Wardener HE, Commentary: salt, blood pressure and health. *Int J Epidemiol* 2002;31:320–327.

3. Ibid.

4. Silver L, Bassett M. Food safety for the 21st century. *JAMA* 2008;300(8):957–959.

5. Most Americans don't understand health effects of wine and sea salt, survey finds. American Heart Association website. Available at: http://newsroom.heart.org/pr/aha/1316.aspx. Accessed February 22, 2012.

6. Bibbins-Domingo K, Chertow GM, Coxson PG, et al. Projected effect of dietary salt reductions on future cardiovascular disease. *N Eng J Med* 2010;362:590–599.

7. U.S. Department of Agriculture and U.S. Department of Health and Human Services. *Dietary Guidelines for Americans, 2010.* Washington, DC: U.S. Government Printing Office; December 2010.

8. Veith I. *Huang Ti Nei Ching Su Wen. The Yellow Emperor's Classic of Internal Medicine.* Baltimore: Williams & Wilkins; 1949. p. 253.

9. Dickinson BD, Havas S, for the Council on Science and Public Health, American Medical Association. Reducing the population burden of cardiovascular disease by reducing sodium intake: a report of the Council on Science and Public Health. *Arch Int Med* 2007;167(14):1460–1468.

10. INTERSALT Cooperative Research Group. INTERSALT: an international study of electrolyte excretion and blood pressure. Results for 24 hour urinary sodium and potassium excretion. *BMJ* 1988;297(6644):319–328.

11. Macgregor GA, Sagnella GA, Markandu ND, Singer DRJ, Cappuccio FP. Double-blind study of three sodium intakes and long-term effects of sodium restriction in essential hypertension. *Lancet* 1989;334:1244–1247.

12. Svetkey LP, Erlinger TP, Vollmer WM, et al. Effect of lifestyle modifications on blood pressure by race, sex, hypertension status, and age. *J Hum Hypertens* 2005;19(1):21–31.

13. Vollmer WM, Sacks FM, Ard J, et al., for the DASH–Sodium Collaborative Research Group. Effects of diet and sodium intake on blood pressure: subgroup analysis of the DASH–Sodium Trial for the DASH–Sodium Trial. *Ann Int Med* 2001;135:1019–1028.

14. Law MR, Frost CD, Wald NJ. By how much does dietary salt reduction lower blood pressure? III—Analysis of data from trials of salt reduction. *BMJ* 1991;302:819–824.

15. Feng JH, MacGregor GA. Effect of modest salt reduction on blood pressure. A meta-analysis of randomized trials: implications for public health. *J Hum Hypertens* 2002;16:761–770.

16. Appel LJ, Brands MW, Daniels SR, et al. Dietary approaches to prevent and treat hypertension: a scientific statement from the American Heart Association. *Hypertens* 2006;47:296–308.

17. Bibbins-Domingo K, Chertow GM, Coxson PG, et al. Projected effect of dietary salt reductions on future cardiovascular disease. *N Eng J Med* 2010;362:590–599.

18. Strazzullo P, Cairella G, Campanozzi A, et al. Population based strategy for dietary salt intake reduction: Italian initiatives in the European framework. *Nutrition, Metabolism & Cardiovascular Disease* 2012;22:161–166.

19. Safar ME, Thuilliez C, Richard V, et al. Pressure-independent contribution of sodium to large artery structure and formation of hypertension. *Cardiovascular Research* 2000;46:269–276.

20. Simon G, Illyes G. High sodium diet induces structural vascular changes in rats without raising blood pressure. *Am J Hypertens* 2000;13(4, Suppl 1):S187.

21. Liebson PR, Grandits G, Prineas R, et al. Echocardiographic correlates of left ventricular structure among 844 mildly hypertensive men and women in the treatment of mild hypertension study (TOMHS). *Circulation* 1993;87:476–486.

22. Perry I, Beevers DG. Salt intake and stroke: a possible direct effect. *J Hum Hypertens* 1992;6(1):23–25.

23. Gow IF, Dockrell M, Edwards CR, et al. The sensitivity of human blood platelets to the aggregating agent ADP during different dietary sodium intakes in healthy men. *Eur J Clin Pharmacol* 1992;43:635–638.

24. Joossens JV, Hill MJ, Elliott P, et al. Dietary salt, nitrate and stomach cancer mortality in 24 countries. European Cancer Prevention (ECP) and the INTERSALT Cooperative Research Group. *Int J Epidemiol* 1996;25(3):494–504.

25. MacGregor GA, Cappuccio FP. The kidney and essential hypertension: a link to osteoporosis. *J Hypertens* 1993;11(8):781–785.

26. Martin TP, Fischer AN. Sodium, potassium, and high blood pressure. *ACSM's Health & Fitness Journal* 2012;16(3):13–21; de Wardener HE, MacGregor GA. Harmful effects of dietary salt in addition to hypertension. *J Hum Hypertens* 2002;16:213–223.

27. Jacobsen, MF. *Salt: The Forgotten Killer*. Washington, DC: Center for Science in the Public Interest; 2005. Available at: http://cspinet .org/new/pdf/salt_report_with_cover.pdf

28. International Food Information Council Foundation. www.foodinsight
    .org/Press-Release/Detail.aspx?topic=Majority_of_Americans_Remain
    _Unaware_and_Unconcerned_About_Sodium_Intake

29. American Heart Association (2011, January 13). Population-wide
    reduction in salt consumption recommended. *ScienceDaily*. Retrieved
    May 28, 2012, from www.sciencedaily.com/releases/2011/01/
    110113213131.htm

30. Danaei G, Ding EL, Mozaffarian D, et al. The preventable causes of
    death in the United States: comparative risk assessment of dietary,
    lifestyle, and metabolic risk factors. *PLoS Medicine* 2009;6(4):1–22.

Chapter Six. Step 3: Eat Bananas

1. Houston MC, Harper KJ. Potassium, magnesium, and calcium: their
   role in both the cause and treatment of hypertension. *J Clin Hypertens* 2008;10(7, Suppl 2):2–11.

2. U.S. Department of Agriculture Center for Nutrition Policy and Promotion. Report of the Dietary Guidelines Advisory Committee on the
   dietary guidelines for Americans, 2010. Available at: www.cnpp.usda
   .gov/dgas2010-dgacreport.htm

3. Appel LJ, Moore TJ, Obarzanek E. A clinical trial of the effects of
   dietary patterns on blood pressure. *N Eng J Med* 1997;336(16):1117–
   1124.

4. Sacks FM, Svetkey LP, Vollmer WM, et al., for the DASH–Sodium
   Collaborative Research Group. Effects on blood pressure of reduced
   dietary sodium and the Dietary Approaches to Stop Hypertension
   (DASH) diet. *N Eng J Med* 2001;344(1):3–10.

5. Appel LJ, Brands MW, Daniels SR, et al. Dietary approaches to prevent and treat hypertension: a scientific statement from the American
   Heart Association. *Hypertens* 2006;47(2):296–308.

6. Institute of Medicine of the National Academies. Dietary reference
   intakes: water, potassium, sodium, chloride and sulfate. www.iom
   .edu/Reports/2004/Dietary-Reference-Intakes-Water-Potassium
   -Sodium-Chloride-and-Sulfate.aspx

7. Grimm RH, Neaton JD, Elmer PJ, et al. The influence of oral potassium chloride on blood pressure in hypertensive men on a low-sodium
   diet. *N Eng J Med* 1990;322(9):623–624.

8. Adrogué HJ, Madias NE. Sodium and potassium in the pathogenesis of hypertension. *N Eng J Med* 2007;356(19):1966–1978.

9. Ward RH, Chin PG, Prior IAM. Tokelau Island migrant study: effect of migration on the familial aggregation of blood pressure. *Hypertens* 1980;2(4):143–154.

10. Krishna GG, Kapoor SC. Potassium depletion exacerbates essential hypertension. *Ann Int Med* 1991;115(2):77–83.

11. D'Elia L, Barba G, Cappuccio FP, Strazzullo P. Potassium intake, stroke, and cardiovascular disease. A meta-analysis of prospective studies. *J Am Coll Cardiol* 2011;57(10):1210–1219.

12. Cook NR, Obarzanek E, Cutler JA, et al., for the Trials of Hypertension Prevention Collaborative Research Group. Joint effects of sodium and potassium intake on subsequent cardiovascular disease: the Trials of Hypertension Prevention follow-up study. *Arch Int Med* 2009;169(1):32–40.

13. INTERSALT Cooperative Research Group. INTERSALT: an international study of electrolyte excretion and blood pressure. Results for 24 hour urinary sodium and potassium excretion. *BMJ* 1988;297(6644):319–328.

14. Adrogué HJ, Madias NE. Sodium and potassium in the pathogenesis of hypertension.

15. Ibid.

16. Appel LJ, Brands MW, Daniels SR, et al. Dietary approaches to prevent and treat hypertension.

Chapter Seven. Step 4: Eat Spinach

1. Sontia B, Touyz RH. Role of magnesium in hypertension. *Archives of Biochemistry and Biophysics* 2007;458:33–39.

2. Chakraborti S, Chakraborti T, Mandal M, et al. Protective role of magnesium in cardiovascular diseases: a review. *Molecular and Cellular Biochemistry* 2002;238:163–179.

3. Rosanoff A, Weaver CM, Rude RK. Suboptimal magnesium status in the United States. Are the health consequences underestimated? *Nutrition Reviews* 2012. Mar;70(3):153–164.

4. Mizushima S, Cappuccio FP, Nichols R, Elliott P. Dietary magnesium intake and blood pressure: a qualitative overview of the observational studies. *J Hum Hypertens* 1998;12(7):447–453.

5. Rosanoff A. Magnesium supplements may enhance the effect of antihypertensive medications in the stage 1 hypertensive subjects. *Magnesium Research* 2010;23(1):27–40.

6. Chobanian AV, Bakris GL, Black HR, et al. The seventh report of the Joint National Committee on Prevention, Detection, Evaluation, and Treatment of High Blood Pressure: the JNC 7 report. *JAMA* 2003;289(19):2560–2571.

7. Jee SH, Miller ER, Guallar F, Singh VK, Appel LJ, Klag MJ. The effect of magnesium supplementation on blood pressure: a meta-analysis of randomized clinical trials. *Am J Hypertens* 2002;15:691–696.

8. Chakraborti S, Chakraborti T, Mandal M, et al. Protective role of magnesium in cardiovascular diseases.

9. Ibid.

10. Paolisso G, Barbagallo M. Hypertension, diabetes mellitus, and insulin resistance. *Am J Hypertens* 1997;10:346–355.

11. Chakraborti S, Chakraborti T, Mandal M, et al. Protective role of magnesium in cardiovascular diseases.

12. Ibid.

13. Song Y, Li TY, van Dam RM, et al. Magnesium intake and plasma markers of systemic inflammation and endothelial dysfunction in women. *Am J Clin Nutr* 2007;85(4):1068–1074.

14. Rosanoff A, Weaver CM, Rude RK. Suboptimal magnesium status in the United States.

Chapter Eight. Step 5: Eat Yogurt

1. Cappuccio FP, Elliott P, Allender PS, Pryer J, Follmann DA, Cutler JA. Epidemiologic association between dietary calcium intake and blood pressure: a meta-analysis of published data. *Am J Epidemiol* 1995;142(9):935–945.

2. Appel L, Moore TJ, Obarzanek E, et al., for the DASH Collaborative

Research Group. A clinical trial of the effects of dietary patterns on blood pressure. *N Eng J Med* 1997;336:1117–1124.

3. McCarron DA, Reusser ME. Finding consensus in the dietary calcium–blood pressure debate. *J Am Coll Nutr* 1999;18(5 Suppl):398S-405S.

4. Heaney RP. Low calcium intake among African Americans: effects on bones and body weight. *J Nutr* 2006;136(4):1095–1098.

5. Appel L, Moore TJ, Obarzanek E, et al, for the DASH Collaborative Research Group. A clinical trial of the effects of dietary patterns on blood pressure.

6. MacMahon S, Peto R, Cutler J, et al. Blood pressure, stroke, and coronary heart disease. Part 1: Prolonged differences in blood pressure: prospective observational studies corrected for the regression dilution bias. *Lancet* 1990;335(8692):765–774.

7. McCarron DA, Reusser ME. Finding consensus in the dietary calcium-blood pressure debate.

8. Griffith LE, Guyatt GH, Cook RJ, et al. The influence of dietary and nondietary calcium supplementation on blood pressure: an updated meta-analysis of randomized controlled trials. *Am J Hypertens* 1999;12:84–92.

9. Allender PS, Cutler JA, Follmann DA, Cappuccio FP, Pryer J, Elliott P. Dietary calcium and blood pressure: a meta-analysis of randomized clinical trials. *Annals Int Med* 1996;124(9):825–831.

10. Bucher HC, Cook RJ, Guyatt GH, et al. Effects of dietary calcium supplementation on blood pressure: a meta-analysis of randomized controlled trials. *JAMA* 1996;275(13):1016–1022.

11. van Mierlo LAJ, Arends LR, Streppel MT, et al. Blood pressure response to calcium supplementation: a meta-analysis of randomized controlled trials. *J Hum Hypertens* (2006);20:571–580. DOI:10.1038/sj.jhh.1002038.

12. van Meijl LEC, Mensink RP. Low-fat dairy consumption reduces systolic blood pressure, but does not improve other metabolic risk parameters in overweight and obese subjects. *Nutr Metabol Cardiovasc Diseases* 2011;21:355–361.

13. Appel L, Moore TJ, Obarzanek E, et al., for the DASH Collaborative Research Group. A clinical trial of the effects of dietary patterns on blood pressure.

14. Bolland MJ, Avenell A, Baron JA, et al. Effect of calcium supplements on risk of myocardial infarction and cardiovascular events: meta-analysis. *BMJ* 2010;29:341:c3691

15. Bolland MJ, Grey A, Avenell A, et al. Calcium supplements with or without vitamin D and risk of cardiovascular events: reanalysis of the Women's Health Initiative limited access dataset and meta-analysis. *BMJ* 2011;342:d2040.

16. LI K, Kaaks R, Linseisen J, et al. Associations of dietary calcium intake and calcium supplementation with myocardial infarction and stroke risk and overall cardiovascular mortality in the Heidelberg cohort of the European Prospective Investigation into Cancer and Nutrition study (EPIC-Heidelberg). *Heart* 2012;98:920–925.

17. Margolis KL, Ray RM, Van Horn L, et al., for the Women's Health Initiative Investigators. Effect of calcium and vitamin D supplementation on blood pressure: the Women's Health Initiative randomized trial. *Hypertens* 2008;52:847–855.

18. Wang L, Manson JE, Buring JE, Lee I-M, Sesso HD. Dietary intake of dairy products, calcium, and vitamin D and the risk of hypertension in middle-aged and older women. *Hypertens* 2008;51:1073–1079.

19. McCarron DA, Reusser ME. Finding consensus in the dietary calcium–blood pressure debate. *J Am Coll Nutr* 1999;18(5):398S–405S.

20. Xu JY, Qin LQ, Wang PY, et al. Effect of milk tripeptides on blood pressure: a meta-analysis of randomized controlled trials. *Nutrition* 2008;24:933–940.

21. Mozaffarian D, Hao T, Rimm EB, et al. Changes in diet and lifestyle and long-term weight gain in women and men. *N Eng J Med* 2011;364:2392–2404.

Chapter Nine. Step 6: Eat Soy

1. Steffen LM, Kroenke CH, Yu X, et al. Associations of plant food, dairy product, and meat intakes with 15–y incidence of elevated blood pressure in young black and white adults: the Coronary Artery Risk Development in Young Adults (CARDIA) study. *Am J Clin Nutr* 2005;82:1169–1177.

2. Pan A, Sun Q, Bernstein AM, et al. Red meat consumption and mortality: results from 2 prospective cohort studies. *Arch Intern Med* 2012;172(7):555–563.

3. Armstrong B, Van Merwyk AJ, Coates H. Blood pressure in Seventh-day Adventist vegetarians. *Am J Epidemiol* 1977;105(5):444–449.

4. Elliott MB, Stamler J, Dyer AR, et al. Association between protein intake and blood pressure: The INTERMAP study. *Arch Intern Med* 2006;166:79–87.

5. Yang G, Shu X-O, Jin F, et al. Longitudinal study of soy food intake and blood pressure among middle-aged and elderly Chinese women. *Am J Clin Nutr* 2005;81:1012–1017.

6. He J, Gu D, Wu X, et al. Effect of soybean protein on blood pressure: a randomized, controlled trial. *Ann Intern Med* 2005;143:1–9.

7. Burke V, Hodgson JM, Beilin LJ, Giangiulioi N, Rodgers P, Puddey IB. Dietary protein and soluble fiber reduce ambulatory BP in treated hypertensives. *Hypertens* 2001;38:821–826.

8. Rivas M, Garay RP, Escanero JF, Cia Jr P, Cia P, Alda JO. Soy milk lowers BP in men and women with mild to moderate essential hypertension. *J Nutr* 2002;132(7):1900–1902.

9. Appel LJ. The effects of protein intake on BP and cardiovascular disease. *Curr Opin Lipidol* 2003;14:55–59.

10. Burke V, Hodgson JM, Beilin LJ, Giangiulioi N, Rodgers P, Puddey IB. Dietary protein and soluble fiber reduce ambulatory BP in treated hypertensives.

11. He J, Gu D, Wu X, et al. Effect of soybean protein on blood pressure.

12. Sagara M, Kanda T, Njelekera M, et al. Effects of dietary intake of soy protein and isoflavones on cardiovascular disease risk factors in high risk, middle-aged men in Scotland. *J Am Coll Nutr* 2003;23(1):85–91.

13. Tsubota-Utsugi M, Ohkubo T, Kikuya M, et al. High fruit intake is associated with a lower risk of future hypertension determined by home blood pressure measurement: the OHASAMA study. *J Hum Hypertens* 2011;25:164–171.

14. McCullough ML, Peterson JL, Patel R, Jacques PF, et al. Flavonoid intake and cardiovascular disease mortality in a prospective cohort of U.S. adults. *Am J Clin Nutr* 2012. DOI:10.3945/ajcn.111.016634.

15. Messina M. Soybean isoflavone exposure does not have feminizing effects on men: a critical examination of the clinical evidence. *Fertil Steril* 2010;93(7):2095–2104.

16. Shu XO, Zheng Y, Cai H, Gu K, Chen Z, Zheng W, Lu W. Soy food intake and breast cancer survival. *JAMA* 2009;302(22):2437–2443.

17. Caan BJ, Natarajan L, Parker BA, Gold EB, Thomson CA, Newman VA, Rock CL, Pu M, Al-Delaimy WK, et al. Soy food consumption and breast cancer prognosis. *Cancer Epidemiol. Biomarkers Prev* 2011;20(5):854–858.

18. Hamilton-Reeves JM, Vazquez G, Duval SJ, Phipps WR, Kurzer MS, Messina MJ. Clinical studies show no effects of soy protein or isoflavones on reproductive hormones in men: results of a meta-analysis. *Fertil Steril* 2010;94(3):997–1007.

19. Messina M, Nagata C, Wu AH. Estimated Asian adult soy protein and isoflavone intakes. *Nutr Cancer* 2006;55(1):1–12.

20. Hamilton-Reeves JM, Vazquez G, Duval SJ, Phipps WR, Kurzer MS, Messina MJ. Clinical studies show no effects of soy protein or isoflavones on reproductive hormones in men.

21. Mitchell JH, Cawood E, Kinniburgh D, Provan A, Collins AR, Irvine DS. Effect of a phytoestrogen food supplement on reproductive health in normal males. *Clin Sci* (Lond) 2001;100:613–618.

22. Beaton LK, McVeigh BL, Dillingham BL, Lampe JW, Duncan AM. Soy protein isolates of varying isoflavone content do not adversely affect semen quality in healthy young men. *Fertil Steril* 2010;94(5):1717–1722.

23. Si H, Liu D. Genistein, a soy phytoestrogen, upregulates the expression of human endothelial nitric oxide synthase and lowers blood pressure in spontaneously hypertensive rats. *J Nutr* 2008;138(2):297–304.

24. Martin D, Song J, Eyster K. Understanding the cardiovascular actions of soy isoflavones: potential novel targets for antihypertensive drug development. *Cardiovascular & Hematological Disorders—Drug Targets* 2008;8(4):297–312.

25. Schmitt CA, Dirsch VM. Modulation of endothelial nitric oxide by plant-derived products. *Nitric Oxide* 2009;21(2):77–91.

26. Woolf KJ, Bisognano JD. Nondrug interventions for treatment of hypertension. *J Clin Hypertens* 2011;13(11):829–835; He J, Gu D, Wu X, et al. Effect of soybean protein on blood pressure.

27. Woolf KJ, Bisognano JD. Nondrug interventions for treatment of hypertension.

28. Nasca MM, Zhou J-R, Welty FK. Effect of soy nuts on adhesion molecules and markers of inflammation in hypertensive and normotensive postmenopausal women. *Am J Cardiol* 2008;102:84–86.

Chapter Ten. Step 7: Eat Dark Chocolate

1. Hollenberg NK, Fisher NDL. Is it the dark in dark chocolate? *Circulation* 2007;116(21):2360–2362.

2. Lee R, Balick MJ, Chocolate: healing food of the gods. *Alternative Therapies in Health and Medicine* 2001;7(5):120–122; Corti R, Flammer AJ, Hollenberg NK, et al. Cocoa and cardiovascular health. *Circulation* 2009;119:1433–1441.

3. Steinberg FM, Bearden MM, Keen CL. Cocoa and chocolate flavonoids: implications for cardiovascular health. *J Am Dietetic Assoc* 2003;103(2):215–223.

4. Grassi D, Lippi C, Pasqualetti P, et al. Short-term administration of flavanol-rich cocoa decreases blood pressure levels and insulin resistance in healthy individuals. *Nutrition, Metabolism & Cardiovascular Diseases* 2004;14(5):294.

5. Hollenberg NK, Fisher NDL. Is it the dark in dark chocolate?

6. Miller KB, et al. Antioxidant activity and polyphenol and procyanidin contents of selected commercially available cocoa-containing and chocolate products in the United States. *J Agr Food Chemistry* 2006;54:4062–4068.

7. Reid K, Sullivan T, Fakler P, et al. Does chocolate reduce blood pressure? A meta-analysis. *BMC Medicine* 2010;8:39; Corti R, Flammer AJ, Hollenberg NK, Lüscher TF. Cocoa and cardiovascular health. *Circulation* 2009;119:1433–1441.

8. Buijsse B, Weikert C, Drogan D, et al. Chocolate consumption in relation to blood pressure and risk of cardiovascular disease in German adults. *Eur Heart J* 2010;31:1616–1623.

9. Buitrago-Lopez A, Sanderson J, Johnson L, et al. Chocolate consumption and cardiometabolic disorders: systemic review and meta-analysis. *BMJ* 2011;343:d4488. DOI:10.1136/bm;.d4488.

10. Grassi D, Lippi C, Pasqualetti P, et al. Short-term administration of flavanol-rich cocoa decreases blood pressure levels and insulin resistance in healthy individuals.

11. Grassi D, Necozione S, Lippi C, et al. Cocoa reduces blood pressure and insulin resistance and improves endothelium-dependent vasodilation in hypertensives. *Hypertens* 2005;46:398–405.

12. Taubert D, Roesen R, Lehmann C, et al. Effects of low habitual cocoa intake on blood pressure and bioactive nitric oxide: a randomized controlled trial. *JAMA* 2007;298(1):49–60.

13. Desch S, Schmidt J, Kobler D, et al. Effect of cocoa products on blood pressure: systematic review and meta-analysis. *Am J Hypertens* 2010;23:97–103.

14. Taubert D, Roesen R, Schömig E. Effect of cocoa and tea intake on blood pressure. *Arch Int Med* 2007;167(7):626–634.

15. Reid K, Sullivan TR, Fakler P, et al. Effect of cocoa on blood pressure. *The Cochrane Library*. Published online: August 15, 2012. DOI:10.1002/14651858.CD008893.pub2.

16. Sánchez O, Quiñones M, et al. Changes in arterial blood pressure of a soluble cocoa fiber product in spontaneously hypertensive rats. *J Agric Food & Food Chem* 2010;58(3):1493–1501.

17. Cienfuegos-Jovellanos E, Quiñones M, Muguerza B, Moulay L, Miguel M, Aleixandre A. Antihypertensive effect of a polyphenol-rich cocoa powder industrially processed to preserve the original flavonoids of the cocoa bean. *J Agric Food & Food Chem* 2009;57(14):6156–6162.

18. Persson IA-L, Persson K, Hagg S, et al. Effects of cocoa extract and dark chocolate on angiotensin-converting enzyme and nitric oxide in human endothelial cells and healthy volunteers. *J Cardiovasc Pharmacol* 2011;57(1):44–50.

19. Galleano M, Oteiza PI, Fraga CG. Cocoa, chocolate, and cardiovascular disease. *J Cardiovasc Pharmacol* 2009;54:483–490.

20. Fisher ND, Hughes M, Gerhard-Herman M, et al. Flavonoid-rich cocoa induces nitric-oxide-dependent vasodilation in healthy humans. *J Hypertens* 2003;21:2281–2286.

21. Heiss C, Kleinbongard P, Dejam A, et al. Acute consumption of flavanol-rich cocoa and the reversal of endothelial dysfunction in smokers. *J Am Coll Cardiol* 2005;46(7):1276–1283.

22. Schroeter H, Heiss C, Balzer J, et al. Epicatechin mediates beneficial effects of flavanol-rich cocoa on vascular function in humans. *Proc Natl Acad Sci USA* 2006;103(4):1024–1029.

23. Di Giuseppe R, Di Castelnuovo A, Centritto F, et al. Regular consumption of dark chocolate is associated with low serum concentrations of C-reactive protein in a healthy Italian population. *J Nutr* 2008;138(10):1939–1945.

24. Galleano M, Oteiza PI, Fraga CG. Cocoa, chocolate, and cardiovascular disease.

25. Miller KB, et al. Antioxidant activity and polyphenol and procyanidin contents of selected commercially available cocoa-containing and chocolate products in the United States. *J Agr Food Chemistry* 2006;54(11):4062–4068.

26. Nieburg O. Industry backs EU call on cocoa child labour and warns 100 percent certified is no guarantee. http://www.confectionerynews .com/Regulation-Safety/Industry-backs-EU-call-on-cocoa-child -labour-and-warns-100-certified-is-no-guarantee

Chapter Eleven. Step 8: Drink Red Wine

1. Forman JP, Stampfer MJ, Curhan GC. Diet and lifestyle risk factors associated with incident hypertension in women. *JAMA* 2009;302(4):401–411.

2. National Institute of Alcohol Abuse and Alcoholism. NIAAA council approves definition of binge drinking. *NIAAA Newsletter* 2004; No. 3, p. 3. Available at: http://pubs.niaaa.nih.gov/publications/Newsletter /winter2004/Newsletter_Number3.pdf

3. Guilford JM, Pezzuto JM. Wine and health: a review. *Am J Enology Viticulture* 2011;62:4.

4. Gaziano JM, Buring JE, Breslow JL, Goldhaber SZ, Rosner B, VanDenburgh M, Willett W, Hennekens CH. Moderate alcohol intake, increased levels of high-density lipoprotein and its subfractions, and decreased risk of myocardial infarction. *N Eng J Med* 1993;329:1829–1834.

5. Zilkens RR, Burke V, Hodgson JM, et al. Red wine and beer elevate blood pressure in normotensive men. *Hypertens* 2005;45: 874–879.

6. Klatsky AL. Alcohol and cardiovascular health. *Physiol Behav* 2010; 100:76–81.

7. Sesso HD, Cook NR, Buring JE, Manson JE, Gaziano JM. Alcohol consumption and the risk of hypertension in women and men. *Hypertens* 2008;51:1080–1087.

8. Stranges S, Wu T, Dorn JM, et al. Relationship of alcohol drinking pattern to risk of hypertension: a population-based study. *Hypertens* 2004;44(6):813–819.

9. Xin X, He J, Frontini MG, Ogden LG, Motsami OI, Whelton PK. Effects of alcohol reduction on blood pressure: a meta-analysis of randomized controlled trials. *Hypertens* 2001;38(5):1112–1117.

10. Witteman JCM, Willett WC, Stampfer MJ, et al. Relation of moderate alcohol consumption and risk of systemic hypertension in women. *Am J Cardiol* 1990;90:633–637.

11. Fuchs FD, Chambless LE, Whelton PK, Nieto FJ, Heiss G. Alcohol consumption and the incidence of hypertension: the atherosclerosis risk in communities study. *Hypertens* 2001;37(5):1242–1250.

12. Stranges S, Wu T, Dorn JM, et al. Relationship of alcohol drinking pattern to risk of hypertension.

13. Malinski MK, Sesso HD, Lopez-Jimenez F, et al. Alcohol consumption and cardiovascular disease mortality in hypertensive men. *Arch Intern Med* 2004;164(6):623–628.

14. Goldberg IJ, Mosca L, Piano MR, et al. Wine and your heart. *Circulation* 2001;103:472–475.

15. Forman JP, Stampfer MJ, Curhan GC. Diet and lifestyle risk factors associated with incident hypertension in women.

16. Bertelli AAA, Das DK. Grapes, wines, resveratrol, and heart health. *J Cardiovasc Pharmacol* 2009;54(6):468–476.

17. Panagiotakos DB, Zeimbekis A, Toutouzas P, et al. The J-shape association of alcohol consumption on blood pressure levels, in elderly people from the Mediterranean islands (MEDIS epidemiological study). *J Hum Hypertens* 2007;21:585–587.

18. Cooper KA, Chopra M, Thurnham DI. Wine polyphenols and promotion of cardiac health. *Nutrition Research Reviews* 2005:17(1):111–129.

19. Bertelli AAA, Das DK. Grapes, wines, resveratrol, and heart health.

20. Waterhouse AL. Wine phenolics. *Annals of the New York Academy of Science* 2002;957(1):21–36.

21. Bertelli AAA, Das DK. Grapes, wines, resveratrol, and heart health.

22. Teragawa H, Fukuda Y, Matsuda K, et al. Effect of alcohol consumption on endothelial function in men with coronary artery disease. *Atherosclerosis* 2002;165(1):145–152.

23. McCullough ML, Peterson JJ, Patel R, et al. Flavonoid intake and cardiovascular disease mortality in a prospective cohort of US adults. *Am J Clin Nutr* 2012;95:454–464.

24. Corder R, Mullen W, Khan NQ, et al. Red wine procyanidins and vascular health. *Nature* 2006;444(7119):566.

25. Gresele P, Pignatelli P, Guglielmini G, et al. Resveratrol, at concentrations attainable with moderate wine consumption, stimulates human platelet nitric oxide production. *J Nutr* 2008;138:1602–1608.

26. Ibid.; Takahashi S, Nakashima Y. Repeated and long-term treatment with physiological concentrations of resveratrol promotes NO production in vascular endothelial cells. *Br J Nutr* 2012;107:774–780.

27. Botden IPG, Langendonk JG, Meima ME, et al. Daily red wine consumption improves vascular function by a soluble guanylyl cyclase-dependent pathway. *Am J Hypertens* 2011;24(2):162–168.

28. Porteri E, Rizzoni D, DeCiuceis C, et al. Vasodilator effects of red wines in subcutaneous small resistance artery of patients with essential hypertension. *Am J Hypertens* 2010;23:373–378.

29. Koppes LLJ, Dekker JM, Hendriks HFJ, et al. Moderate alcohol consumption lowers risk of type 2 diabetes. *Diabetes Care* 2005;28(3):719–725.

30. Freiberg M, Cabral HJ, Heeren TC, et al. Alcohol consumption and the prevalence of the metabolic syndrome in the US: A cross-sectional analysis of data from the National Health and Nutrition Examination Survey. *Diabetes Care* 2004;27(11):2954–2959.

31. Chiva-Blanch G, Urpi-Sarda M, Llorach R, et al. Differential effects of polyphenols and alcohol of red wine on the expression of adhesion molecules and inflammatory cytokine related to atherosclerosis: a randomized clinical trial. *Am J Clin Nutr* 2012. DOI:10.3945/ajcn.111.022889.

32. Kwon JY, Seo SG, Heo YS, et al. Piceatannol, natural polypheno-
lic stillbene, inhibits adipogenesis via modulation of mitotic clonal
expansion and insulin receptor-dependent insulin signaling in early
phase of differentiation. *J Biol Chem* 2012;287(14):11566–11578.

Chapter Twelve. Step 9: Take Four Supplements

1. Kim DH, Sabour S, Sagar UN, et al. Prevalence of hypovita-
minosis D in cardiovascular disease (from the National Health
and Nutrition Examination Survey 2001 to 2004). *Am J Cardiol*
2008;102(11):1540–1544.

2. Wu SH, Ho SC, Zhong L. Effects of vitamin D supplementation on
blood pressure. *SMJ* 2010;103(8):729–737.

3. Mayer Jr O, Filopovsky J, Seidlerova J, et al. The association between
low 25-hydroxyvitamin D and increased aortic stiffness. *J Hum Hypertens* 2012;(11):650–655.

4. Wu SH, Ho SC, Zhong L. Effects of vitamin D supplementation on
blood pressure.

5. Li YC. Vitamin D regulation of the renin-angiotensin system. *J Cellular Biochem* 2003;88(2):327–331.

6. Woolf KJ, Bisognano JD. Nondrug interventions for treatment of
hypertension. *J Clin Hypertens* 2011;13(11):829–835.

7. Tripkovic L, Lambert H, Hart K, et al. Comparison of vitamin D_2
and vitamin D_3 supplementation in raising serum 25-hydroxyvita-
min D status: a systematic review and meta-analysis. *Am J Clin Nutr*
2012;95:1357–1364.

8. Yamagami T, Shibata N, Folkers K. Bioenergetics in clinical medicine.
Studies on coenzyme Q_{10} and essential hypertension. *Res Commun
Chem Pathol Pharmacol* 1975;11:273–288.

9. Rosenfeldt FL, Haas SJ, Krum H, et al. Coenzyme Q_{10} in the treatment of hypertension: a meta-analysis of the clinical trials. *J Hum
Hypertens* 2007;21(4):297–306.

10. Young JM, Florkowski CM, Molyneux SL, et al. A randomized,
double-blind, placebo-controlled crossover study of coenzyme Q_{10}
therapy in hypertensive patients with the metabolic syndrome. *Am J
Hypertens* 2012;25(2):261–270.

11. Rosenfeldt FL, Haas SJ, Krum H, et al. Coenzyme Q_{10} in the treatment of hypertension.

12. Gebauer SK, Psota TL, Harris WS, et al. n-3 fatty acid dietary recommendations and food sources to achieve essentiality and cardiovascular benefits. *Am J Clin Nutr* 2006;83(Suppl):1526S–1535S.

13. Geleijnse JM, Giltay EJ, Grobbee DE, et al. Blood pressure response to fish oil supplementation: metaregression analysis of randomized trials. *J Hypertens* 2002;20:1493–1499.

14. Pase MP, Grima NA, Sarris J. The effects of dietary and nutrient interventions on arterial stiffness: a systematic review. *Am J Clin Nutr* 2011. Feb;93:446–454.

15. Wang Q, Liang X, Wang L, et al. Effect of omega-3 fatty acids supplementation on endothelial function: a meta-analysis of randomized controlled trials. *Atherosclerosis* 2012;221:536–543.

16. Larsson SC, Virtamo J, Wolk A. Fish consumption and risk of stroke in Swedish women. *Am J Clin Nutr* 2011;93:487–493.

17. Reinders JK, Virtanen IA, Brower T-P, et al. Association of serum n-3 polyunsaturated fatty acids with C-reactive protein in men. *Eur J Clin Nutr*. Advance online publication: November 23, 2011. DOI:10.1038/ejcn.2011.195.

18. Mori TA, Burke V, Puddey IB, et al. Effect of fish diets and weight loss on serum leptin concentration in overweight, treated hypertensive subjects. *J Hypertens* 2004;22(10):1983–1990.

19. Ueshima H, Stamler J, Elliott P, et al. Food omega-3 fatty acid intake of individuals (total, linoleic acid, long-chain) and their blood pressure INTERMAP study. *Hypertens* 2007;50:313–319; Shay CM, Stamler J, Dyer AR, et al. Nutrient and food intakes of middle-aged adults at low risk of cardiovascular disease: the international study of macro-/micronutrients and blood pressure (INTERMAP). *Eur J Nutr* 2011. DOI:10.1007/s00394-011-0268-2.

20. Woolf KJ, Bisognano JD. Nondrug interventions for treatment of hypertension.

Chapter Thirteen. Step 10: Exercise

1. Roger VL, Go AS, Lloyd-Jones DM, Benjamin EJ, et al., on behalf of the American Heart Association Statistics Committee and Stroke

Statistics Subcommittee. Heart disease and stroke statistics—2012 update: a report from the American Heart Association. *Circulation* 2012;125:e2–e220.

2. Pescatello LS, Guidry MA, Blanchard BE, et al. Exercise intensity alters postexercise hypotension. *J Hypertens* 2004;22:1881–1888.

3. Ibid.

4. Physical Activity Guidelines Advisory Committee. *Physical Activity Guidelines Advisory Committee Report, 2008*. Washington, DC: U.S. Department of Health and Human Services; 2008.

5. Whelton SP, Chin A, Xin X, He J. Effect of aerobic exercise on blood pressure: a meta-analysis of randomized, controlled trials. *Ann Int Med* 2002;136:493–503.

6. Fagard RH. Exercise characteristics and the blood pressure response to dynamic physical training. *Medicine Science Sports & Exercise* 2001;33(6):S484–S492.

7. Pescatello LS, Franklin BA, Fagard R, Farquhar WB, Kelley GA, Ray CA. Exercise and hypertension: American College of Sports Medicine position stand. *Med Sci Sports* 2004;36(3):533–552.

8. Physical Activity Guidelines Advisory Committee. *Physical Activity Guidelines Advisory Committee Report, 2008*.

9. Nualnim N, Parkhurst K, Dhindsa M, et al. Effect of swimming training on blood pressure and vascular function in adults > 50 years of age. *Am J Cardiol* 2012;109:1005–1010.

10. Pescatello LS, Guidry MA, Blanchard BE, et al. Exercise intensity alters postexercise hypotension.

11. Cornelissen VA, Verheyden B, Aubert AE, Fagard RH. Effects of aerobic training intensity on resting, exercise and post-exercise blood pressure, heart rate and heart-rate variability. *J Hum Hypertens* 2010;24(3):175–182.

12. Tsutsumi A, Kayaha K, Kario K, et al. Prospective study on occupational stress and risk of stroke. *Arch Intern Med* 2009;169(1):56–61.

13. Truelsen T, Nielsen N, Boysen G, et al. Self-reported stress and risk of stroke: the Copenhagen city heart study. *Stroke* 2003;34:856–862.

14. Khan N, Hemmelgarn B, Padwal R, et al. The 2009 Canadian Hypertension Education Program recommendations for the management of hypertension: part 2—therapy. *Can J Cardiol* 2009;25(5):287–298.

15. Dickinson HO, Campbell F, Beyer FR, et al. Relaxation therapies for the management of primary hypertension in adults: a Cochrane review. *J Hum Hypertens* 2008;22(12):809–820.

16. Mourya M, Mahajan AS, Singh NP, Jain AK. Effect of slow- and fast-paced breathing exercises on autonomic functions in patients with essential hypertension. *J Altern Complementary Med* 2009;15(7):711–717.

17. Okonta NR. Does yoga therapy reduce blood pressure in patients with hypertension? *Holistic Nurse Practitioner* 2012;26(3):137–141.

18. Andersen JW, Liu C, Kryscio RJ. Blood pressure response to transcendental meditation: a meta-analysis. *Am J Hypertension* 2008;21: 310–316.

19. Rainforth MV, Schneider RH, Nidich SI, Gaylord-King C, Salerno JW, Anderson JW. Stress reduction programs in patients with elevated blood pressure: a systematic review and meta-analysis. *Curr Hypertens Rep* 2007;9(6):520–528.

20. Schneider RH, Alexander CN, Staggers F, et al. Long-term effects of stress reduction on mortality in persons ≥55 years of age with systemic hypertension. *Am J Cardiol* 2005;95:1060–1064.

21. Joseph CN, Porta C, Casucci G, et al. Slow breathing improves arterial baroflex sensitivity and decreases blood pressure in essential hypertension. *Hypertens* 2005;46:714–718.

22. Manikonda JP, Störk S, Tögel S, et al. Contemplative meditation reduces ambulatory blood pressure and stress-induced hypertension: a randomized pilot trial. *J Hum Hypertens* 2008;22(2):138–140.

23. Zaros P, Romero Pires CEM, Bacci Jr M, et al. Effect of 6 months of physical exercise on the nitrate/nitrite levels in hypertensive postmenopausal women. *BMC Women's Health* 2009:9(17). DOI:10.1186/1472-6874-9-17.

24. Bobik A, Grassi G. Low-grade inflammation and arterial stiffness in the elderly. *J Hypertens* 2012;30:679–681.

25. Van Craenenbroeck EM, Conraads VM. Mending injured endothelium in chronic heart failure: a new target for exercise training. *Int J Cardiol* 2012. DOI:10.1016/j.ijcard.2012.04.106.

26. Mourya M, Mahajan AS, Singh NP, Jain AK. Effect of slow- and fast-paced breathing exercises on autonomic functions in patients with essential hypertension.

A Few Closing Words from Dr. Janet

1. Committee on Public Health Priorities to Reduce and Control Hypertension in the U.S. Population; Board on Population Health and Public Health Practice. *A Population-Based Policy and Systems Change Approach to Prevent and Control Hypertension.* Washington, DC: Institute of Medicine of the National Academies Press; 2010.

Index

About the Author

JANET BOND BRILL grew up in New York City, the daughter of a prominent actor and a psychoanalyst. She graduated from the Walden School in Manhattan and earned a B.S. in biology, as well as both a master's degree and a doctoral degree in exercise physiology, at the University of Miami. She also holds a second master's degree in nutrition science from Florida International University. She is a registered dietitian, certified personal trainer, and certified wellness coach.

Dr. Brill is the author of *Cholesterol Down* and *Prevent a Second Heart Attack,* and she has also been published in noted scientific journals, including the *International Journal of Sport Nutrition,* the *International Journal of Obesity,* and the *American Journal of Lifestyle Medicine,* as well as published and quoted in leading consumer publications, including *Shape, Prevention,* and *Men's Health.*

She is a frequent professional speaker, a nutrition expert on national television, and maintains a private nutrition consulting practice. Dr. Brill also serves as director of nutrition for Fitness Together Franchise Corporation, the world's largest business of personal trainers.

Dr. Brill practices what she preaches, having completed four marathons and countless road races, many for charitable causes. Dr. Brill enjoys spending her free time with her husband, Sam; her three children; and her three dogs, Simba, Bentley, and Pippa.

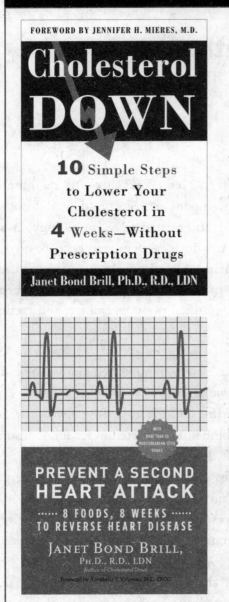